AF797168

Wine Tasting Journal

Dedication

I dedicate this book to all of my wine lovers out there who need a places to jot down and recored the good, the bad and the ugly of the wines you have experienced.

With Love,

-L. Bracey

Introductions

I created this journal for all of you wine lovers out there to have a place to write done the wines you taste along this journey called life.

Sometimes along our journey we come across some unforgettable wines, this journal is designed for you to have an actual account of the experience, the taste and how you rate the wine.

Wheather your at home, out on the town, or you've stumbled upon some quaint little vineyard write down your wines and keep an account of your experiences.

-L Bracey

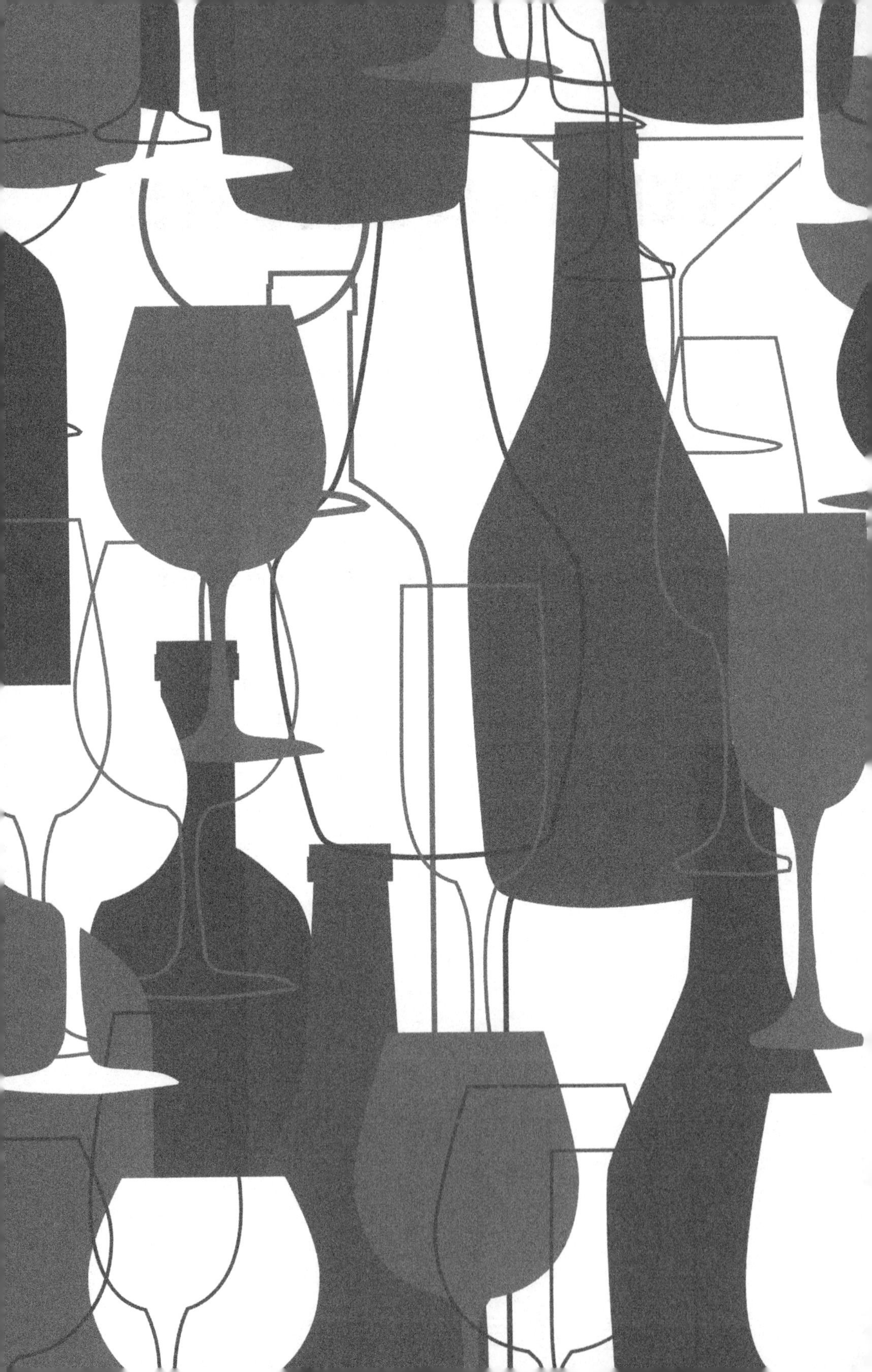

Wine: ______________________ Date Tasted: __________

Region/Country: ______________________

Grape: ______________________

% Alcohol: ______________________

Producer: ______________ Vintage: ______________

Importer/Distributor: ______________

Price: ______________

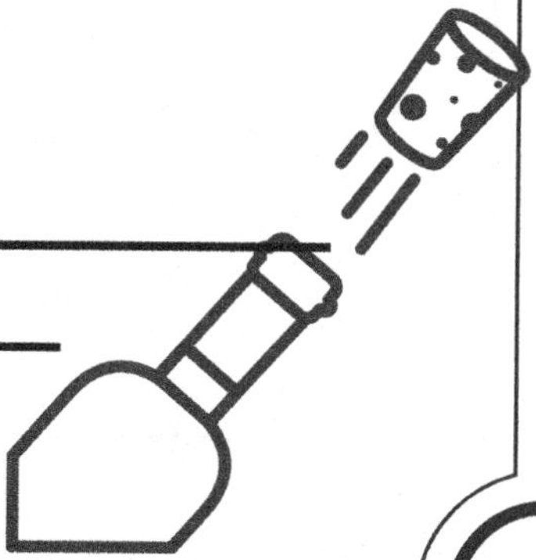

Color/Style: Red White Rose' Sparkling Effervescent Fortified

Appearance: Thin Thick

Dry/Sweet Spectrum: Dry 1 2 3 4 5 6 7 8 9 10 Sweet

Body: Light Light to Medium Medium Medium to Full Full Overall

Tasting Experience: Poor 1 2 3 4 5 6 7 8 9 10 Excellent

Comments:

____

____

____

____

Recommended Not Recommended

Circle One

Wine: ______________________ Date Tasted: __________

Region/Country: ______________________

Grape: ______________________

% Alcohol: ______________________

Producer: ____________ Vintage: ____________

Importer/Distributor: ______________

Price: ____________

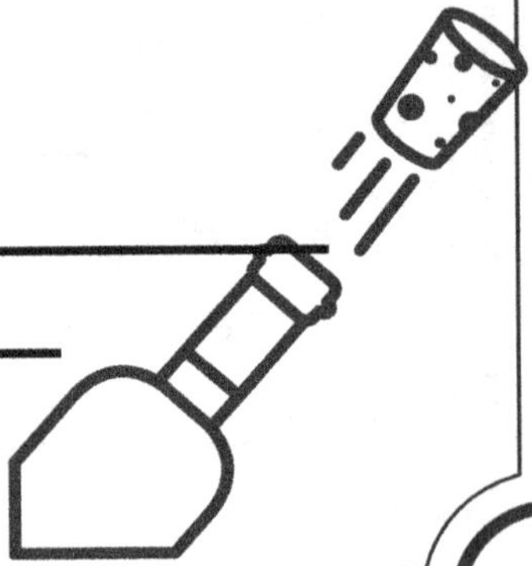

Color/Style: Red White Rose' Sparkling Effervescent Fortified
Appearance: Thin Thick
Dry/Sweet Spectrum: Dry 1 2 3 4 5 6 7 8 9 10 Sweet
Body: Light Light to Medium Medium Medium to Full Full Overall
Tasting Experience: Poor 1 2 3 4 5 6 7 8 9 10 Excellent

Comments:

____

____

____

____

Recommended Not Recommended

Circle One

Wine: ______________________ Date Tasted: __________

Region/Country: ______________________

Grape: ______________________

% Alcohol: ______________________

Producer: ______________ Vintage: ______________

Importer/Distributor: ______________

Price: ______________

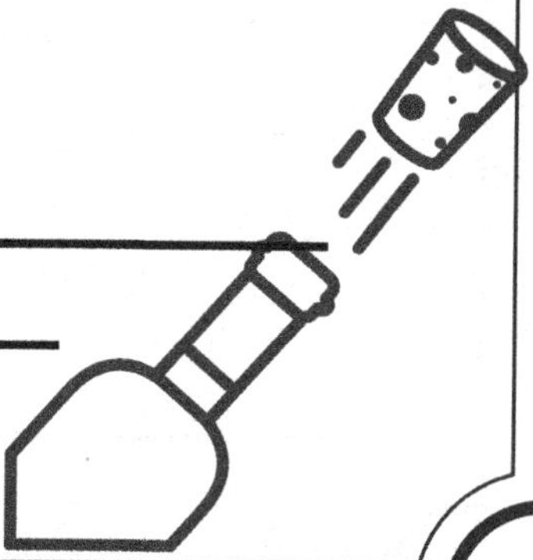

Color/Style: Red White Rose' Sparkling Effervescent Fortified

Appearance: Thin Thick

Dry/Sweet Spectrum: Dry 1 2 3 4 5 6 7 8 9 10 Sweet

Body: Light Light to Medium Medium Medium to Full Full Overall

Tasting Experience: Poor 1 2 3 4 5 6 7 8 9 10 Excellent

Comments:

____

____

____

____

Recommended Not Recommended

Circle One

Wine: ____________________ Date Tasted: __________

Region/Country: ____________________

Grape: ____________________

% Alcohol: ____________________

Producer: ____________ Vintage: ____________

Importer/Distributor: ____________

Price: ____________

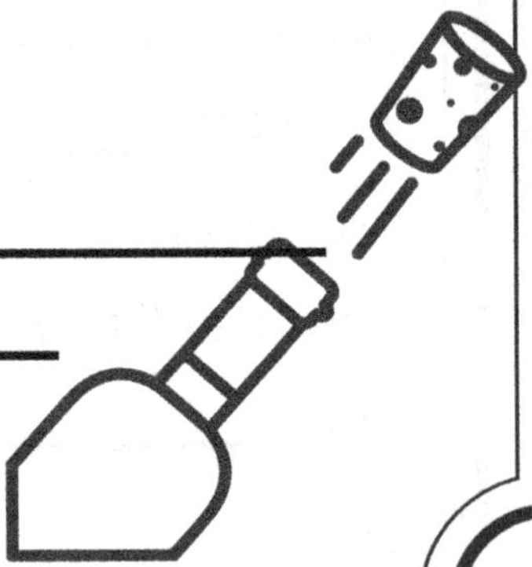

Color/Style: Red White Rose' Sparkling Effervescent Fortified

Appearance: Thin Thick

Dry/Sweet Spectrum: Dry 1 2 3 4 5 6 7 8 9 10 Sweet

Body: Light Light to Medium Medium Medium to Full Full Overall

Tasting Experience: Poor 1 2 3 4 5 6 7 8 9 10 Excellent

Comments:

Recommended Not Recommended

Circle One

Wine: ____________________ Date Tasted: __________

Region/Country: ____________________

Grape: ____________________

% Alcohol: ____________________

Producer: ____________ Vintage: ____________

Importer/Distributor: ____________

Price: ____________

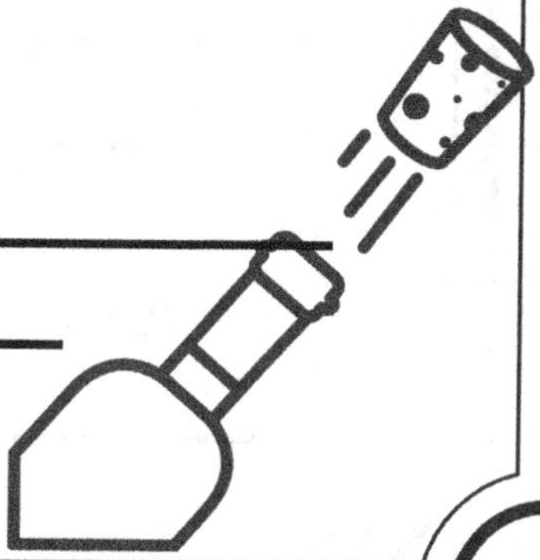

Color/Style: Red White Rose' Sparkling Effervescent Fortified

Appearance: Thin Thick

Dry/Sweet Spectrum: Dry 1 2 3 4 5 6 7 8 9 10 Sweet

Body: Light Light to Medium Medium Medium to Full Full Overall

Tasting Experience: Poor 1 2 3 4 5 6 7 8 9 10 Excellent

Comments:

Recommended Not Recommended

Circle One

Wine: ____________________ Date Tasted: __________

Region/Country: ____________________

Grape: ____________________

% Alcohol: ____________________

Producer: ____________ Vintage: ____________

Importer/Distributor: ____________

Price: ____________

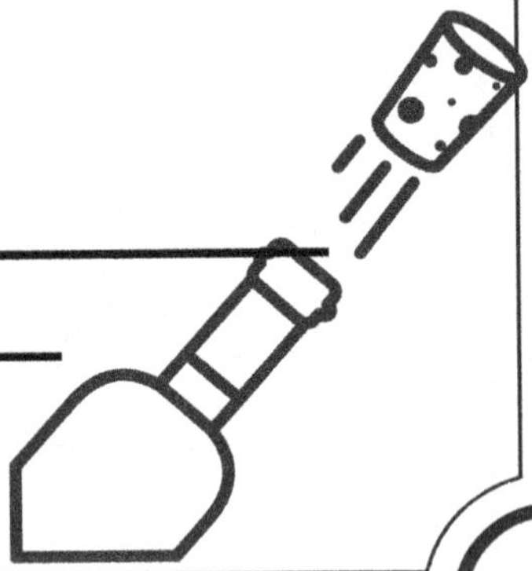

Color/Style: Red White Rose' Sparkling Effervescent Fortified

Appearance: Thin Thick

Dry/Sweet Spectrum: Dry 1 2 3 4 5 6 7 8 9 10 Sweet

Body: Light Light to Medium Medium Medium to Full Full Overall

Tasting Experience: Poor 1 2 3 4 5 6 7 8 9 10 Excellent

Comments:

Recommended Not Recommended

Circle One

Wine: ______________________ Date Tasted: __________

Region/Country: ______________________

Grape: ______________________

% Alcohol: ______________________

Producer: ______________ Vintage: ______________

Importer/Distributor: ______________

Price: ______________

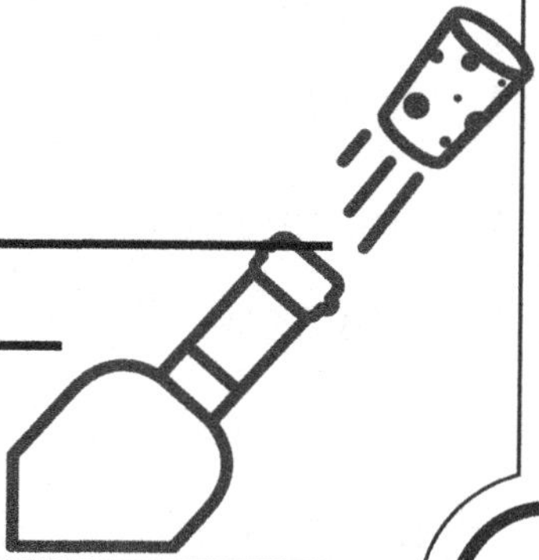

Color/Style: Red White Rose' Sparkling Effervescent Fortified

Appearance: Thin Thick

Dry/Sweet Spectrum: Dry 1 2 3 4 5 6 7 8 9 10 Sweet

Body: Light Light to Medium Medium Medium to Full Full Overall

Tasting Experience: Poor 1 2 3 4 5 6 7 8 9 10 Excellent

Comments:

____

____

____

____

Recommended Not Recommended

Circle One

Wine: ____________ Date Tasted: ________

Region/Country: ____________

Grape: ____________

% Alcohol: ____________

Producer: ________ Vintage: ________

Importer/Distributor: ________

Price: ________

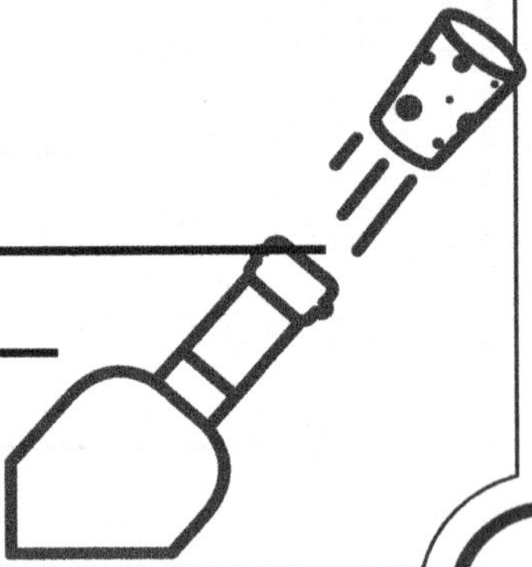

Color/Style: Red White Rose' Sparkling Effervescent Fortified

Appearance: Thin Thick

Dry/Sweet Spectrum: Dry 1 2 3 4 5 6 7 8 9 10 Sweet

Body: Light Light to Medium Medium Medium to Full Full Overall

Tasting Experience: Poor 1 2 3 4 5 6 7 8 9 10 Excellent

Comments:

____

____

____

____

Recommended Not Recommended

Circle One

Wine: ______________ Date Tasted: ________

Region/Country: ______________

Grape: ______________

% Alcohol: ______________

Producer: __________ Vintage: __________

Importer/Distributor: __________

Price: __________

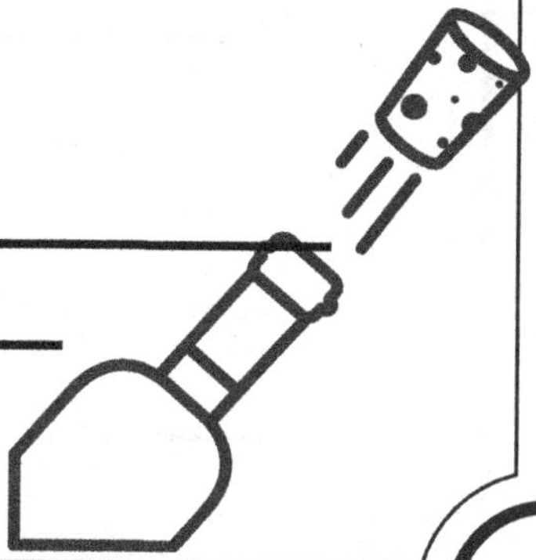

Color/Style: Red White Rose' Sparkling Effervescent Fortified

Appearance: Thin Thick

Dry/Sweet Spectrum: Dry 1 2 3 4 5 6 7 8 9 10 Sweet

Body: Light Light to Medium Medium Medium to Full Full Overall

Tasting Experience: Poor 1 2 3 4 5 6 7 8 9 10 Excellent

Comments:

____

____

____

____

Recommended Not Recommended

Circle One

Wine: ____________________ Date Tasted: __________

Region/Country: ____________________

Grape: ____________________

% Alcohol: ____________________

Producer: ____________ Vintage: ____________

Importer/Distributor: ____________

Price: ____________

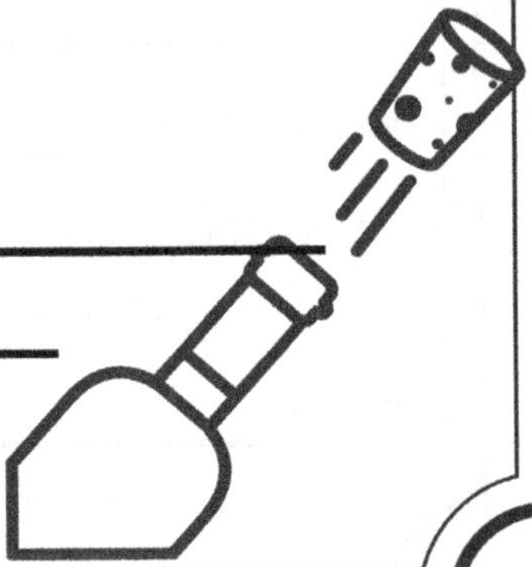

Color/Style: Red White Rose' Sparkling Effervescent Fortified

Appearance: Thin Thick

Dry/Sweet Spectrum: Dry 1 2 3 4 5 6 7 8 9 10 Sweet

Body: Light Light to Medium Medium Medium to Full Full Overall

Tasting Experience: Poor 1 2 3 4 5 6 7 8 9 10 Excellent

Comments:

____

____

____

____

Recommended Not Recommended

Circle One

Wine: ____________ Date Tasted: ________

Region/Country: ____________

Grape: ____________

% Alcohol: ____________

Producer: ________ Vintage: ________

Importer/Distributor: ________

Price: ________

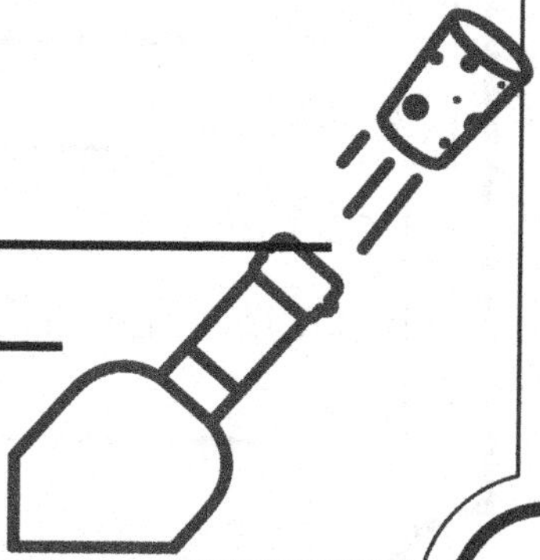

Color/Style: Red White Rose' Sparkling Effervescent Fortified

Appearance: Thin Thick

Dry/Sweet Spectrum: Dry 1 2 3 4 5 6 7 8 9 10 Sweet

Body: Light Light to Medium Medium Medium to Full Full Overall

Tasting Experience: Poor 1 2 3 4 5 6 7 8 9 10 Excellent

Comments:

____

____

____

____

Recommended Not Recommended

Circle One

Wine: ____________ Date Tasted: ________

Region/Country: ____________

Grape: ____________

% Alcohol: ____________

Producer: ________ Vintage: ________

Importer/Distributor: ________

Price: ________

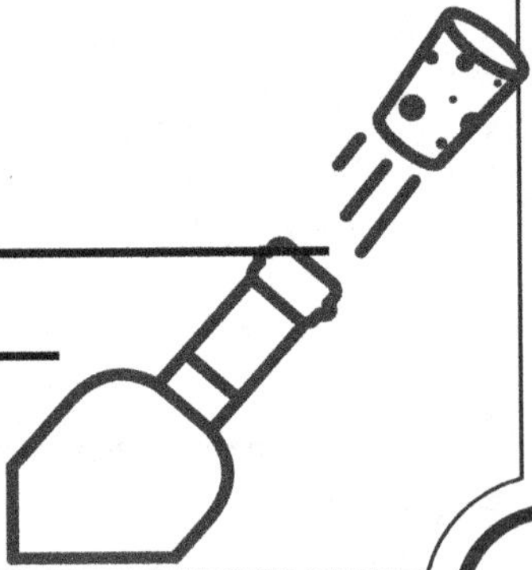

Color/Style: Red White Rose' Sparkling Effervescent Fortified

Appearance: Thin Thick

Dry/Sweet Spectrum: Dry 1 2 3 4 5 6 7 8 9 10 Sweet

Body: Light Light to Medium Medium Medium to Full Full Overall

Tasting Experience: Poor 1 2 3 4 5 6 7 8 9 10 Excellent

Comments:

Recommended Not Recommended

Circle One

Wine: ____________________ Date Tasted: ________

Region/Country: ____________________

Grape: ____________________

% Alcohol: ____________________

Producer: ____________ Vintage: ____________

Importer/Distributor: ____________

Price: ____________

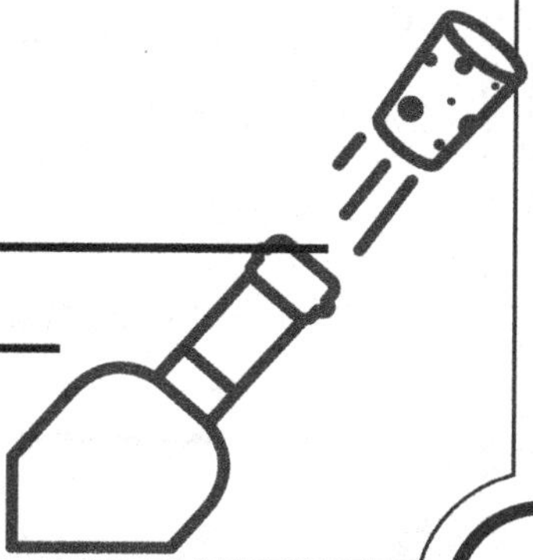

Color/Style: Red White Rose' Sparkling Effervescent Fortified

Appearance: Thin Thick

Dry/Sweet Spectrum: Dry 1 2 3 4 5 6 7 8 9 10 Sweet

Body: Light Light to Medium Medium Medium to Full Full Overall

Tasting Experience: Poor 1 2 3 4 5 6 7 8 9 10 Excellent

Comments:

____

____

____

____

Recommended Not Recommended

Circle One

Wine: ______________________ Date Tasted: __________

Region/Country: ______________________

Grape: ______________________

% Alcohol: ______________________

Producer: ____________ Vintage: ____________

Importer/Distributor: ____________

Price: ____________

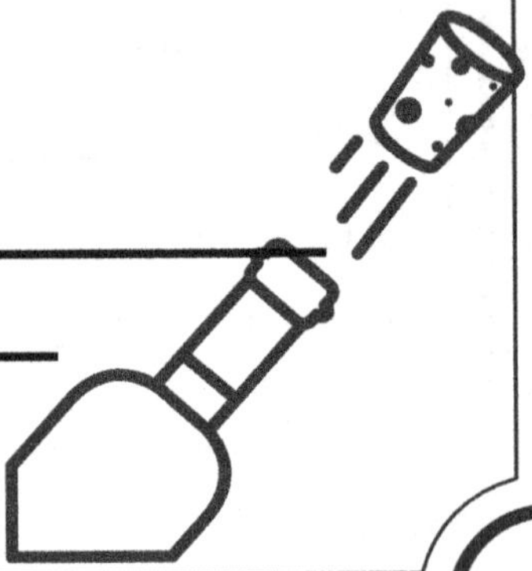

Color/Style: Red White Rose' Sparkling Effervescent Fortified

Appearance: Thin Thick

Dry/Sweet Spectrum: Dry 1 2 3 4 5 6 7 8 9 10 Sweet

Body: Light Light to Medium Medium Medium to Full Full Overall

Tasting Experience: Poor 1 2 3 4 5 6 7 8 9 10 Excellent

Comments:

____

____

____

____

Recommended Not Recommended

Circle One

Wine: ________________ Date Tasted: ________

Region/Country: ________________

Grape: ________________

% Alcohol: ________________

Producer: __________ Vintage: __________

Importer/Distributor: __________

Price: __________

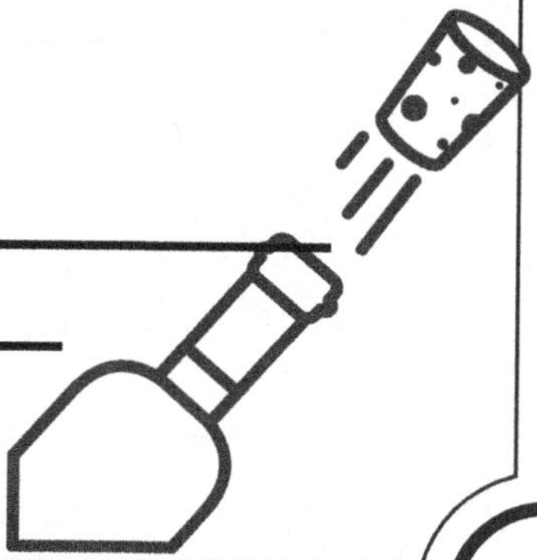

Color/Style: Red White Rose' Sparkling Effervescent Fortified

Appearance: Thin Thick

Dry/Sweet Spectrum: Dry 1 2 3 4 5 6 7 8 9 10 Sweet

Body: Light Light to Medium Medium Medium to Full Full Overall

Tasting Experience: Poor 1 2 3 4 5 6 7 8 9 10 Excellent

Comments:

Recommended Not Recommended

Circle One

Wine: ________________ Date Tasted: ________

Region/Country: ________________

Grape: ________________

% Alcohol: ________________

Producer: __________ Vintage: __________

Importer/Distributor: __________

Price: __________

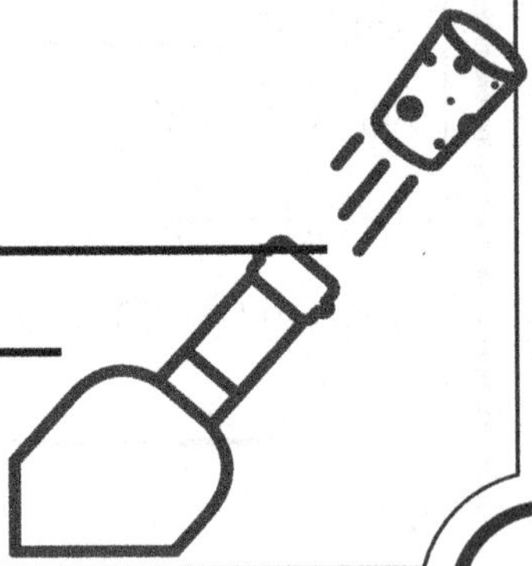

Color/Style: Red White Rose' Sparkling Effervescent Fortified

Appearance: Thin Thick

Dry/Sweet Spectrum: Dry 1 2 3 4 5 6 7 8 9 10 Sweet

Body: Light Light to Medium Medium Medium to Full Full Overall

Tasting Experience: Poor 1 2 3 4 5 6 7 8 9 10 Excellent

Comments:

Recommended Not Recommended

Circle One

Wine: ________________ Date Tasted: ________

Region/Country: ________________

Grape: ________________

% Alcohol: ________________

Producer: __________ Vintage: __________

Importer/Distributor: __________

Price: __________

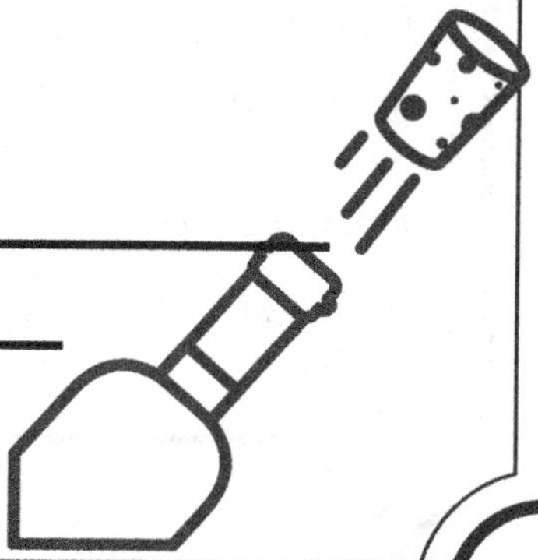

Color/Style: Red White Rose' Sparkling Effervescent Fortified

Appearance: Thin Thick

Dry/Sweet Spectrum: Dry 1 2 3 4 5 6 7 8 9 10 Sweet

Body: Light Light to Medium Medium Medium to Full Full Overall

Tasting Experience: Poor 1 2 3 4 5 6 7 8 9 10 Excellent

Comments:

____

____

____

____

Recommended Not Recommended

Circle One

Wine: ____________________ Date Tasted: __________

Region/Country: ____________________

Grape: ____________________

% Alcohol: ____________________

Producer: ____________ Vintage: ____________

Importer/Distributor: ____________

Price: ____________

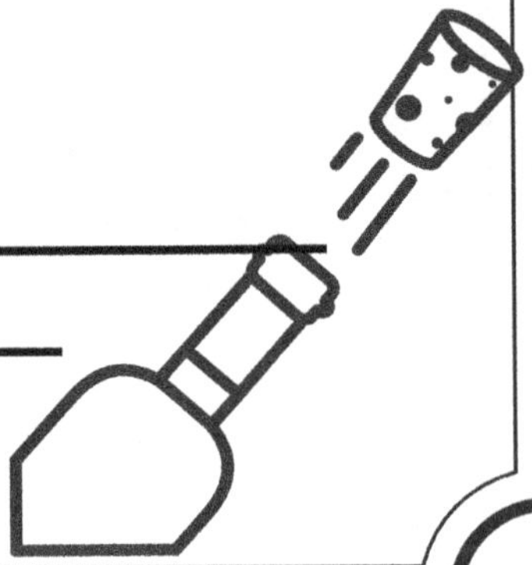

Color/Style: Red White Rose' Sparkling Effervescent Fortified

Appearance: Thin Thick

Dry/Sweet Spectrum: Dry 1 2 3 4 5 6 7 8 9 10 Sweet

Body: Light Light to Medium Medium Medium to Full Full Overall

Tasting Experience: Poor 1 2 3 4 5 6 7 8 9 10 Excellent

Comments:

____

____

____

____

Recommended Not Recommended

Circle One

Wine: ______________ Date Tasted: ________

Region/Country: ______________

Grape: ______________

% Alcohol: ______________

Producer: __________ Vintage: __________

Importer/Distributor: __________

Price: __________

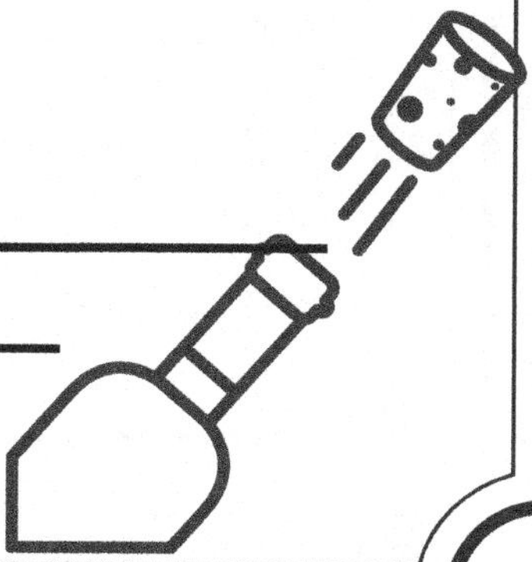

Color/Style: Red White Rose' Sparkling Effervescent Fortified

Appearance: Thin Thick

Dry/Sweet Spectrum: Dry 1 2 3 4 5 6 7 8 9 10 Sweet

Body: Light Light to Medium Medium Medium to Full Full Overall

Tasting Experience: Poor 1 2 3 4 5 6 7 8 9 10 Excellent

Comments:

____

____

____

____

Recommended Not Recommended

Circle One

Wine: ____________ Date Tasted: ________

Region/Country: ____________

Grape: ____________

% Alcohol: ____________

Producer: ________ Vintage: ________

Importer/Distributor: ________

Price: ________

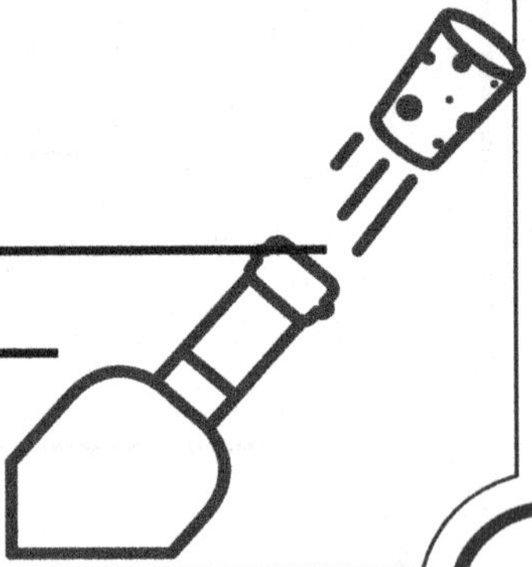

Color/Style: Red White Rose' Sparkling Effervescent Fortified

Appearance: Thin Thick

Dry/Sweet Spectrum: Dry 1 2 3 4 5 6 7 8 9 10 Sweet

Body: Light Light to Medium Medium Medium to Full Full Overall

Tasting Experience: Poor 1 2 3 4 5 6 7 8 9 10 Excellent

Comments:

____

____

____

____

Recommended Not Recommended

Circle One

Wine: ____________________ Date Tasted: __________

Region/Country: ____________________

Grape: ____________________

% Alcohol: ____________________

Producer: ____________ Vintage: ____________

Importer/Distributor: ____________

Price: ____________

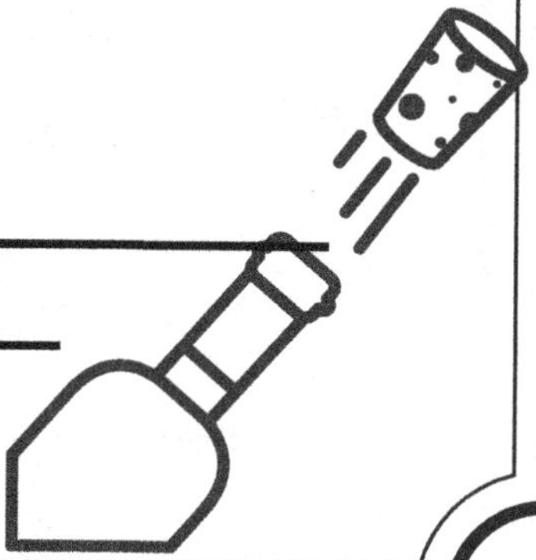

Color/Style: Red White Rose' Sparkling Effervescent Fortified

Appearance: Thin Thick

Dry/Sweet Spectrum: Dry 1 2 3 4 5 6 7 8 9 10 Sweet

Body: Light Light to Medium Medium Medium to Full Full Overall

Tasting Experience: Poor 1 2 3 4 5 6 7 8 9 10 Excellent

Comments:

Recommended Not Recommended

Circle One

Wine: ____________________ Date Tasted: ________

Region/Country: ____________________

Grape: ____________________

% Alcohol: ____________________

Producer: ____________ Vintage: ____________

Importer/Distributor: ____________

Price: ____________

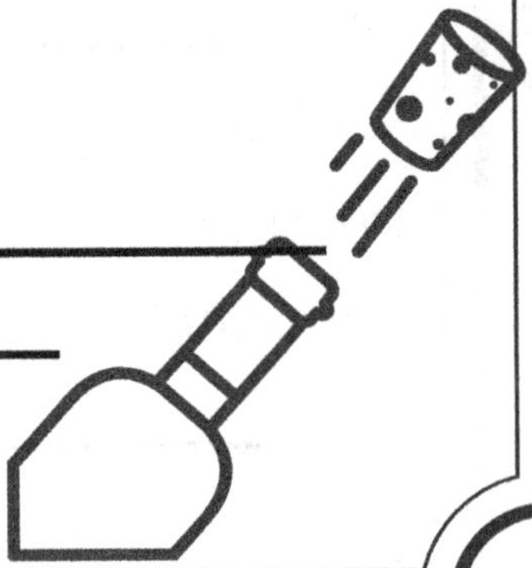

Color/Style: Red White Rose' Sparkling Effervescent Fortified

Appearance: Thin Thick

Dry/Sweet Spectrum: Dry 1 2 3 4 5 6 7 8 9 10 Sweet

Body: Light Light to Medium Medium Medium to Full Full Overall

Tasting Experience: Poor 1 2 3 4 5 6 7 8 9 10 Excellent

Comments:

____

____

____

____

Recommended Not Recommended

Circle One

Wine: ____________________ Date Tasted: __________

Region/Country: ____________________

Grape: ____________________

% Alcohol: ____________________

Producer: ____________ Vintage: ____________

Importer/Distributor: ____________

Price: ____________

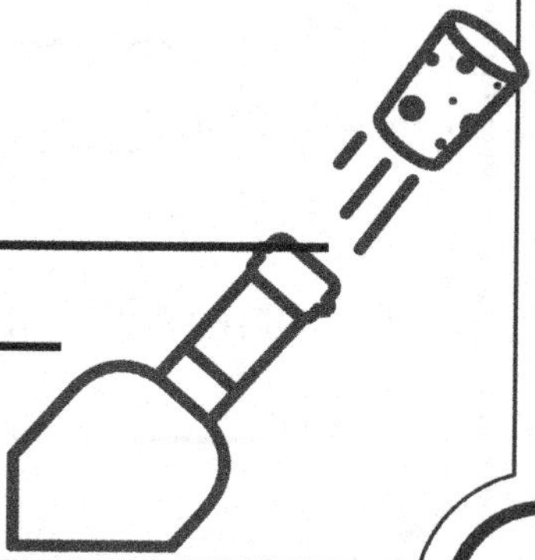

Color/Style: Red White Rose' Sparkling Effervescent Fortified

Appearance: Thin Thick

Dry/Sweet Spectrum: Dry 1 2 3 4 5 6 7 8 9 10 Sweet

Body: Light Light to Medium Medium Medium to Full Full Overall

Tasting Experience: Poor 1 2 3 4 5 6 7 8 9 10 Excellent

Comments:

____

____

____

____

Recommended Not Recommended

Circle One

Wine: ____________________ Date Tasted: __________

Region/Country: ____________________

Grape: ____________________

% Alcohol: ____________________

Producer: ____________ Vintage: ____________

Importer/Distributor: ____________

Price: ____________

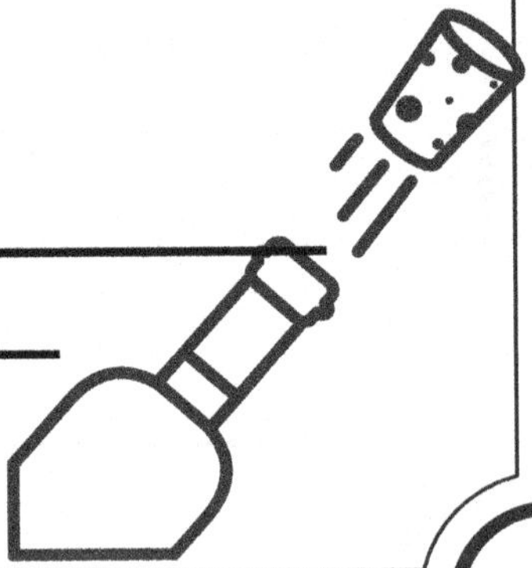

Color/Style: Red White Rose' Sparkling Effervescent Fortified

Appearance: Thin Thick

Dry/Sweet Spectrum: Dry 1 2 3 4 5 6 7 8 9 10 Sweet

Body: Light Light to Medium Medium Medium to Full Full Overall

Tasting Experience: Poor 1 2 3 4 5 6 7 8 9 10 Excellent

Comments:

Recommended Not Recommended

Circle One

Wine: ________________ Date Tasted: _______

Region/Country: ________________

Grape: ________________

% Alcohol: ________________

Producer: __________ Vintage: __________

Importer/Distributor: __________

Price: __________

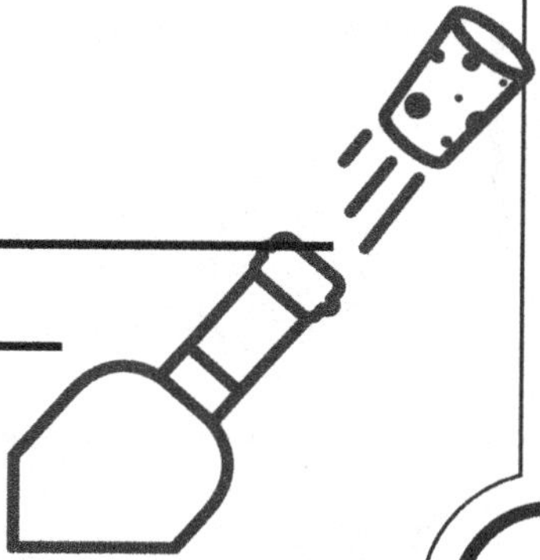

Color/Style: Red White Rose' Sparkling Effervescent Fortified

Appearance: Thin Thick

Dry/Sweet Spectrum: Dry 1 2 3 4 5 6 7 8 9 10 Sweet

Body: Light Light to Medium Medium Medium to Full Full Overall

Tasting Experience: Poor 1 2 3 4 5 6 7 8 9 10 Excellent

Comments:

Recommended Not Recommended

Circle One

Wine: ______________________ Date Tasted: __________

Region/Country: ______________________

Grape: ____________________

% Alcohol: ______________________

Producer: ____________ Vintage: ____________

Importer/Distributor: ______________

Price: ______________

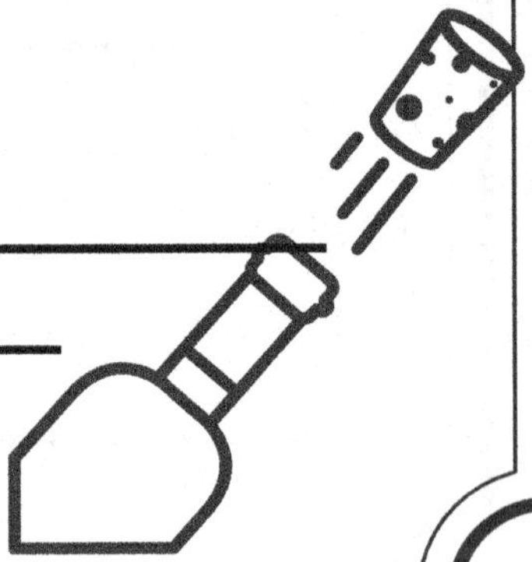

Color/Style: Red White Rose' Sparkling Effervescent Fortified

Appearance: Thin Thick

Dry/Sweet Spectrum: Dry 1 2 3 4 5 6 7 8 9 10 Sweet

Body: Light Light to Medium Medium Medium to Full Full Overall

Tasting Experience: Poor 1 2 3 4 5 6 7 8 9 10 Excellent

Comments:

____

____

____

____

Recommended Not Recommended

Circle One

Wine: ____________________ Date Tasted: __________

Region/Country: ____________________

Grape: ____________________

% Alcohol: ____________________

Producer: ____________ Vintage: ____________

Importer/Distributor: ____________

Price: ____________

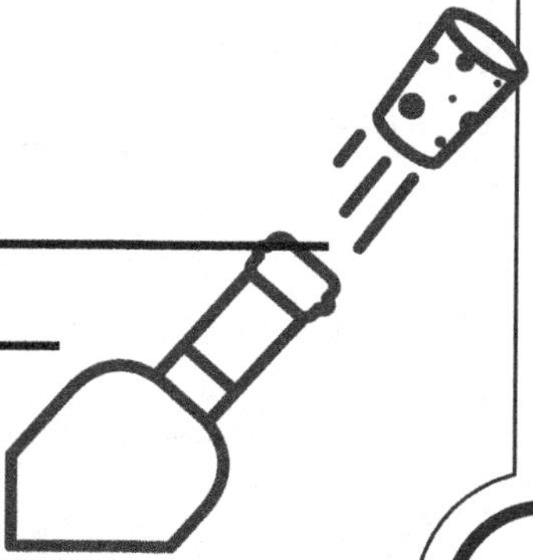

Color/Style: Red White Rose' Sparkling Effervescent Fortified

Appearance: Thin Thick

Dry/Sweet Spectrum: Dry 1 2 3 4 5 6 7 8 9 10 Sweet

Body: Light Light to Medium Medium Medium to Full Full Overall

Tasting Experience: Poor 1 2 3 4 5 6 7 8 9 10 Excellent

Comments:

____

____

____

____

Recommended Not Recommended

Circle One

Wine: ____________ Date Tasted: ________

Region/Country: ____________

Grape: ____________

% Alcohol: ____________

Producer: ________ Vintage: ________

Importer/Distributor: ________

Price: ________

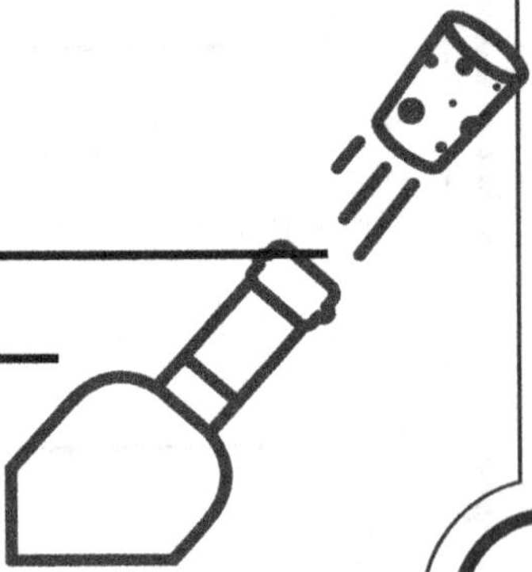

Color/Style: Red White Rose' Sparkling Effervescent Fortified

Appearance: Thin Thick

Dry/Sweet Spectrum: Dry 1 2 3 4 5 6 7 8 9 10 Sweet

Body: Light Light to Medium Medium Medium to Full Full Overall

Tasting Experience: Poor 1 2 3 4 5 6 7 8 9 10 Excellent

Comments:

Recommended Not Recommended

Circle One

Wine: ______________________ Date Tasted: __________

Region/Country: ______________________

Grape: ______________________

% Alcohol: ______________________

Producer: ______________ Vintage: ______________

Importer/Distributor: ______________

Price: ______________

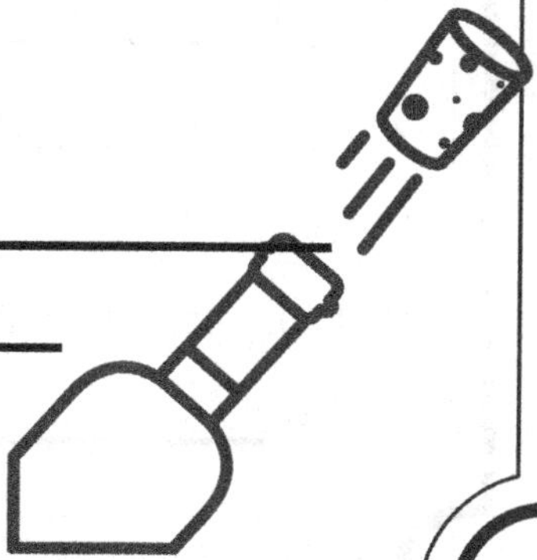

Color/Style: Red White Rose' Sparkling Effervescent Fortified

Appearance: Thin Thick

Dry/Sweet Spectrum: Dry 1 2 3 4 5 6 7 8 9 10 Sweet

Body: Light Light to Medium Medium Medium to Full Full Overall

Tasting Experience: Poor 1 2 3 4 5 6 7 8 9 10 Excellent

Comments:

____

____

____

____

Recommended Not Recommended

Circle One

Wine: ____________________ Date Tasted: ________

Region/Country: ____________________

Grape: ____________________

% Alcohol: ____________________

Producer: ____________ Vintage: ____________

Importer/Distributor: ____________

Price: ____________

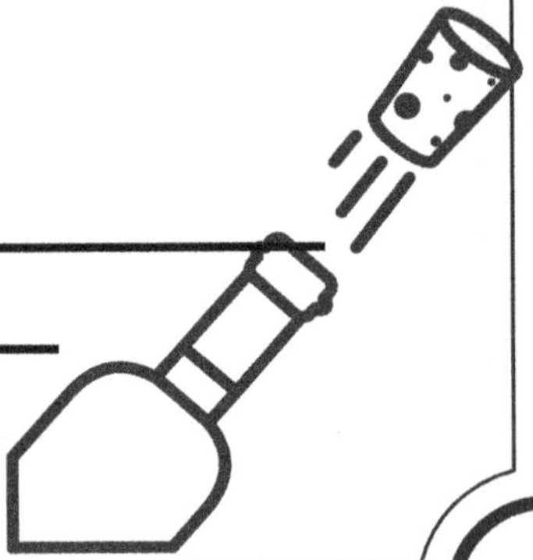

Color/Style: Red White Rose' Sparkling Effervescent Fortified

Appearance: Thin Thick

Dry/Sweet Spectrum: Dry 1 2 3 4 5 6 7 8 9 10 Sweet

Body: Light Light to Medium Medium Medium to Full Full Overall

Tasting Experience: Poor 1 2 3 4 5 6 7 8 9 10 Excellent

Comments:

Recommended Not Recommended

Circle One

Wine: ____________ Date Tasted: ________

Region/Country: ____________

Grape: ____________

% Alcohol: ____________

Producer: ________ Vintage: ________

Importer/Distributor: ________

Price: ________

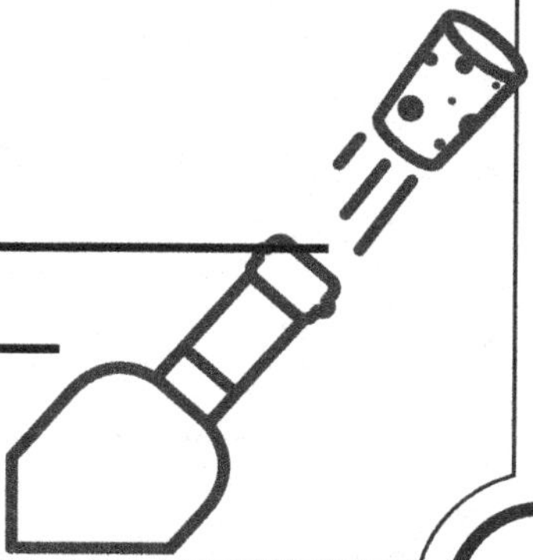

Color/Style: Red White Rose' Sparkling Effervescent Fortified

Appearance: Thin Thick

Dry/Sweet Spectrum: Dry 1 2 3 4 5 6 7 8 9 10 Sweet

Body: Light Light to Medium Medium Medium to Full Full Overall

Tasting Experience: Poor 1 2 3 4 5 6 7 8 9 10 Excellent

Comments:

____

____

____

____

Recommended Not Recommended

Circle One

Wine: ______________ Date Tasted: ______

Region/Country: ______________

Grape: ______________

% Alcohol: ______________

Producer: __________ Vintage: __________

Importer/Distributor: __________

Price: __________

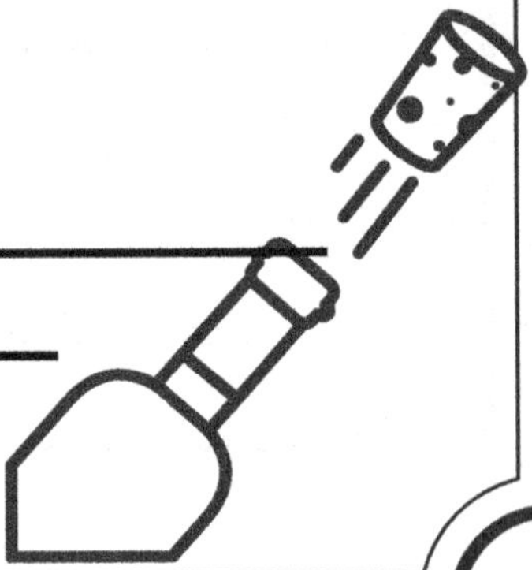

Color/Style: Red White Rose' Sparkling Effervescent Fortified

Appearance: Thin Thick

Dry/Sweet Spectrum: Dry 1 2 3 4 5 6 7 8 9 10 Sweet

Body: Light Light to Medium Medium Medium to Full Full Overall

Tasting Experience: Poor 1 2 3 4 5 6 7 8 9 10 Excellent

Comments:

____

____

____

____

Recommended Not Recommended

Circle One

Wine: ____________________ Date Tasted: __________

Region/Country: ____________________

Grape: ____________________

% Alcohol: ____________________

Producer: ____________ Vintage: ____________

Importer/Distributor: ____________

Price: ____________

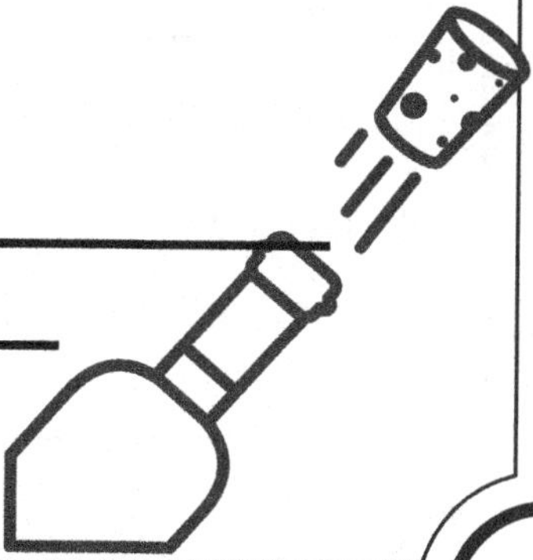

Color/Style: Red White Rose' Sparkling Effervescent Fortified

Appearance: Thin Thick

Dry/Sweet Spectrum: Dry 1 2 3 4 5 6 7 8 9 10 Sweet

Body: Light Light to Medium Medium Medium to Full Full Overall

Tasting Experience: Poor 1 2 3 4 5 6 7 8 9 10 Excellent

Comments:

____

____

____

____

Recommended Not Recommended

Circle One

Wine: ____________________ Date Tasted: __________

Region/Country: ____________________

Grape: ____________________

% Alcohol: ____________________

Producer: ____________ Vintage: ____________

Importer/Distributor: ____________

Price: ____________

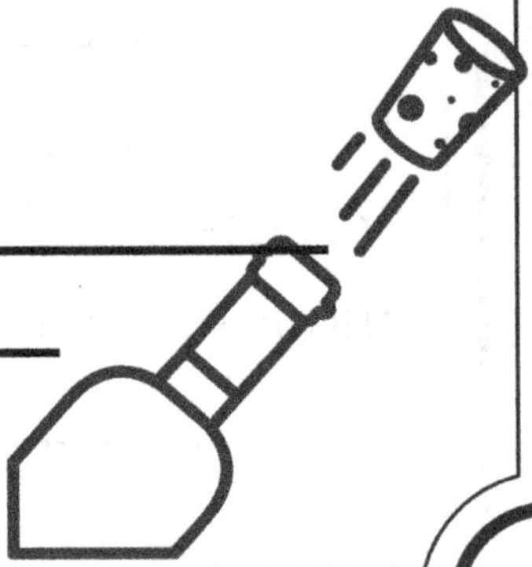

Color/Style: Red White Rose' Sparkling Effervescent Fortified

Appearance: Thin Thick

Dry/Sweet Spectrum: Dry 1 2 3 4 5 6 7 8 9 10 Sweet

Body: Light Light to Medium Medium Medium to Full Full Overall

Tasting Experience: Poor 1 2 3 4 5 6 7 8 9 10 Excellent

Comments:

____

____

____

____

Recommended Not Recommended

Circle One

Wine: ____________________ Date Tasted: __________

Region/Country: ____________________

Grape: ____________________

% Alcohol: ____________________

Producer: ____________ Vintage: ____________

Importer/Distributor: ____________

Price: ____________

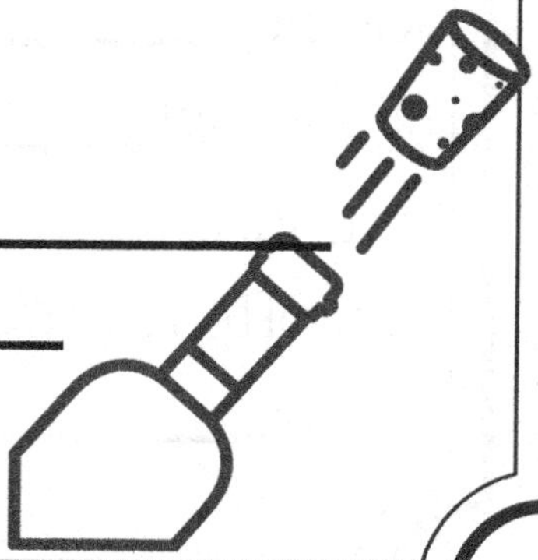

Color/Style: Red White Rose' Sparkling Effervescent Fortified

Appearance: Thin Thick

Dry/Sweet Spectrum: Dry 1 2 3 4 5 6 7 8 9 10 Sweet

Body: Light Light to Medium Medium Medium to Full Full Overall

Tasting Experience: Poor 1 2 3 4 5 6 7 8 9 10 Excellent

Comments:

____

____

____

____

Recommended Not Recommended

Circle One

Wine: ____________________ Date Tasted: __________

Region/Country: ____________________

Grape: ____________________

% Alcohol: ____________________

Producer: ____________ Vintage: ____________

Importer/Distributor: ____________

Price: ____________

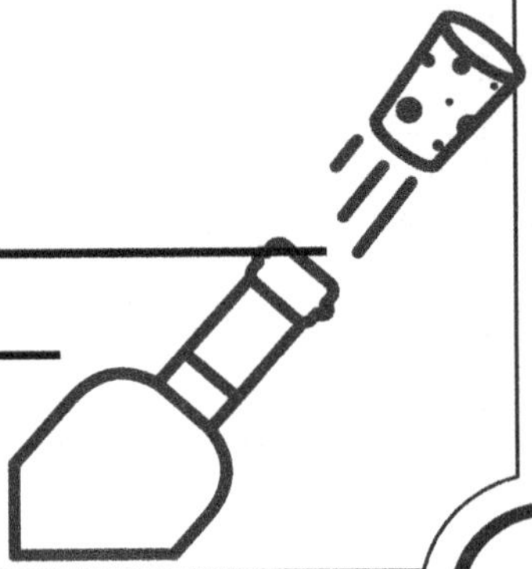

Color/Style: Red White Rose' Sparkling Effervescent Fortified

Appearance: Thin Thick

Dry/Sweet Spectrum: Dry 1 2 3 4 5 6 7 8 9 10 Sweet

Body: Light Light to Medium Medium Medium to Full Full Overall

Tasting Experience: Poor 1 2 3 4 5 6 7 8 9 10 Excellent

Comments:

____

____

____

____

Recommended Not Recommended

Circle One

Wine: ________________ Date Tasted: ________

Region/Country: ________________

Grape: ________________

% Alcohol: ________________

Producer: __________ Vintage: __________

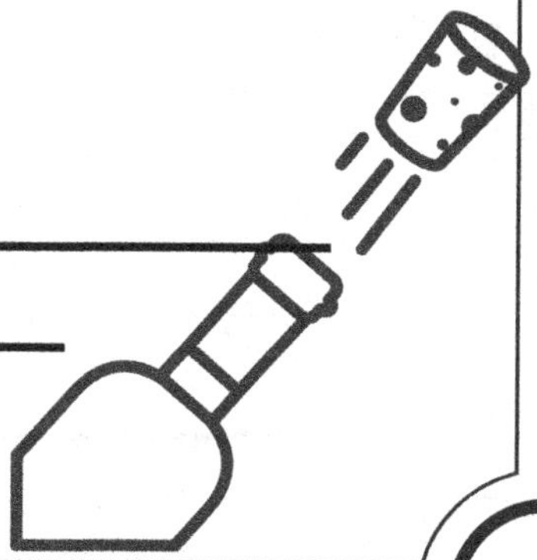

Importer/Distributor: __________

Price: __________

Color/Style: Red White Rose' Sparkling Effervescent Fortified

Appearance: Thin Thick

Dry/Sweet Spectrum: Dry 1 2 3 4 5 6 7 8 9 10 Sweet

Body: Light Light to Medium Medium Medium to Full Full Overall

Tasting Experience: Poor 1 2 3 4 5 6 7 8 9 10 Excellent

Comments:

____

____

____

____

Recommended Not Recommended

Circle One

Wine: ____________________ Date Tasted: ________

Region/Country: ____________________

Grape: ____________________

% Alcohol: ____________________

Producer: ____________ Vintage: ____________

Importer/Distributor: ____________

Price: ____________

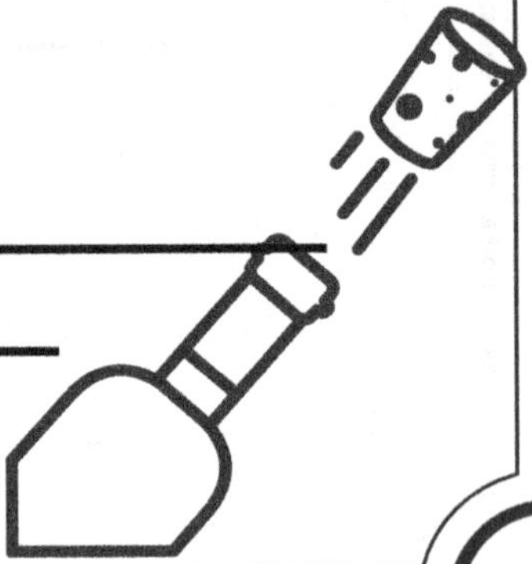

Color/Style: Red White Rose' Sparkling Effervescent Fortified

Appearance: Thin Thick

Dry/Sweet Spectrum: Dry 1 2 3 4 5 6 7 8 9 10 Sweet

Body: Light Light to Medium Medium Medium to Full Full Overall

Tasting Experience: Poor 1 2 3 4 5 6 7 8 9 10 Excellent

Comments:

____

____

____

____

Recommended Not Recommended

Circle One

Wine: ____________________ Date Tasted: ________

Region/Country: ____________________

Grape: ____________________

% Alcohol: ____________________

Producer: ____________ Vintage: ____________

Importer/Distributor: ____________

Price: ____________

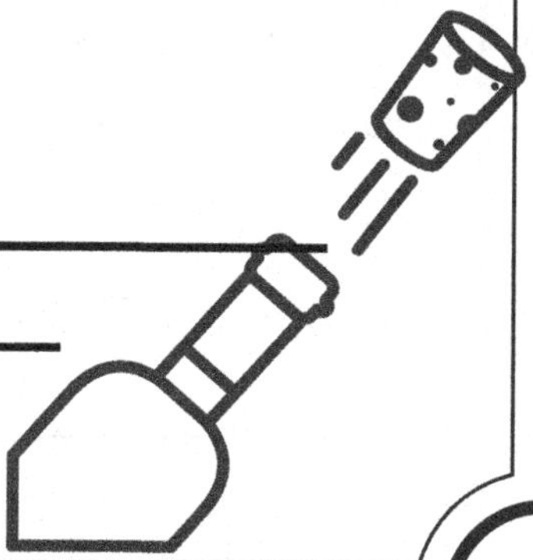

Color/Style: Red White Rose' Sparkling Effervescent Fortified

Appearance: Thin Thick

Dry/Sweet Spectrum: Dry 1 2 3 4 5 6 7 8 9 10 Sweet

Body: Light Light to Medium Medium Medium to Full Full Overall

Tasting Experience: Poor 1 2 3 4 5 6 7 8 9 10 Excellent

Comments:

____

____

____

____

Recommended Not Recommended

Circle One

Wine: ______________________ Date Tasted: __________

Region/Country: ______________________

Grape: ______________________

% Alcohol: ______________________

Producer: ______________ Vintage: ______________

Importer/Distributor: ______________

Price: ______________

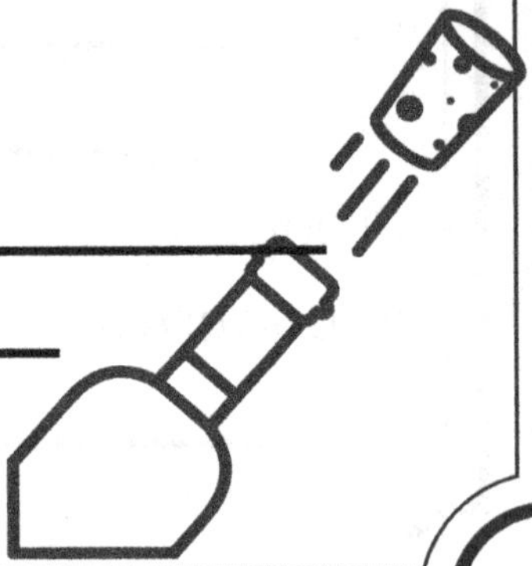

Color/Style: Red White Rose' Sparkling Effervescent Fortified

Appearance: Thin Thick

Dry/Sweet Spectrum: Dry 1 2 3 4 5 6 7 8 9 10 Sweet

Body: Light Light to Medium Medium Medium to Full Full Overall

Tasting Experience: Poor 1 2 3 4 5 6 7 8 9 10 Excellent

Comments:

Recommended Not Recommended

Circle One

Wine: ____________ Date Tasted: ________

Region/Country: ____________

Grape: ____________

% Alcohol: ____________

Producer: ________ Vintage: ________

Importer/Distributor: ________

Price: ________

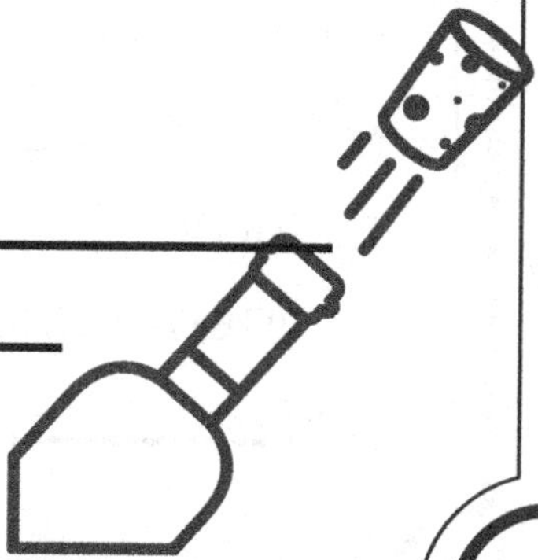

Color/Style: Red White Rose' Sparkling Effervescent Fortified

Appearance: Thin Thick

Dry/Sweet Spectrum: Dry 1 2 3 4 5 6 7 8 9 10 Sweet

Body: Light Light to Medium Medium Medium to Full Full Overall

Tasting Experience: Poor 1 2 3 4 5 6 7 8 9 10 Excellent

Comments:

____

____

____

____

Recommended Not Recommended

Circle One

Wine: ____________ Date Tasted: ________

Region/Country: ____________

Grape: ____________

% Alcohol: ____________

Producer: ________ Vintage: ________

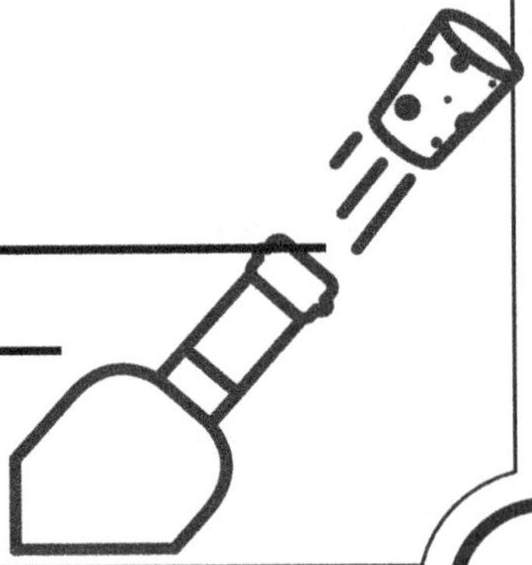

Importer/Distributor: ________

Price: ________

Color/Style: Red White Rose' Sparkling Effervescent Fortified
Appearance: Thin Thick
Dry/Sweet Spectrum: Dry 1 2 3 4 5 6 7 8 9 10 Sweet
Body: Light Light to Medium Medium Medium to Full Full Overall
Tasting Experience: Poor 1 2 3 4 5 6 7 8 9 10 Excellent

Comments:

____

____

____

____

Recommended Not Recommended

Circle One

Wine: ________________ Date Tasted: ________

Region/Country: ________________

Grape: ________________

% Alcohol: ________________

Producer: ____________ Vintage: ____________

Importer/Distributor: ____________

Price: ____________

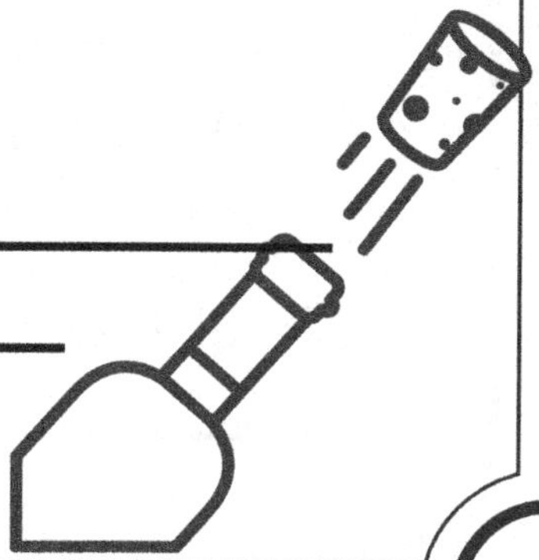

Color/Style: Red White Rose' Sparkling Effervescent Fortified

Appearance: Thin Thick

Dry/Sweet Spectrum: Dry 1 2 3 4 5 6 7 8 9 10 Sweet

Body: Light Light to Medium Medium Medium to Full Full Overall

Tasting Experience: Poor 1 2 3 4 5 6 7 8 9 10 Excellent

Comments:

____

____

____

____

Recommended Not Recommended

Circle One

Wine: ____________________ Date Tasted: __________

Region/Country: ____________________

Grape: ____________________

% Alcohol: ____________________

Producer: ____________ Vintage: ____________

Importer/Distributor: ____________

Price: ____________

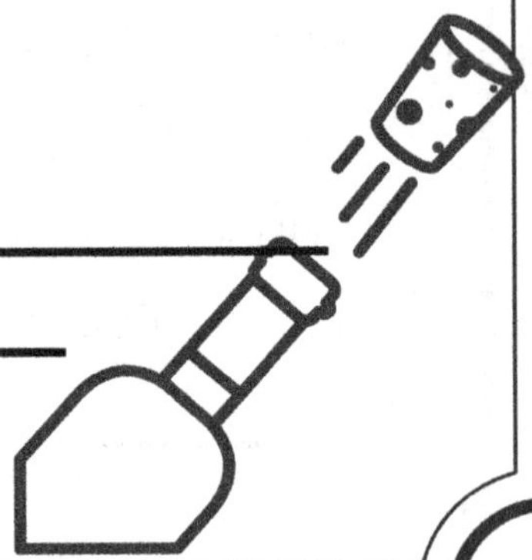

Color/Style: Red White Rose' Sparkling Effervescent Fortified

Appearance: Thin Thick

Dry/Sweet Spectrum: Dry 1 2 3 4 5 6 7 8 9 10 Sweet

Body: Light Light to Medium Medium Medium to Full Full Overall

Tasting Experience: Poor 1 2 3 4 5 6 7 8 9 10 Excellent

Comments:

Recommended Not Recommended

Circle One

Wine: ____________________ Date Tasted: ________

Region/Country: ____________________

Grape: ____________________

% Alcohol: ____________________

Producer: ____________ Vintage: ____________

Importer/Distributor: ____________

Price: ____________

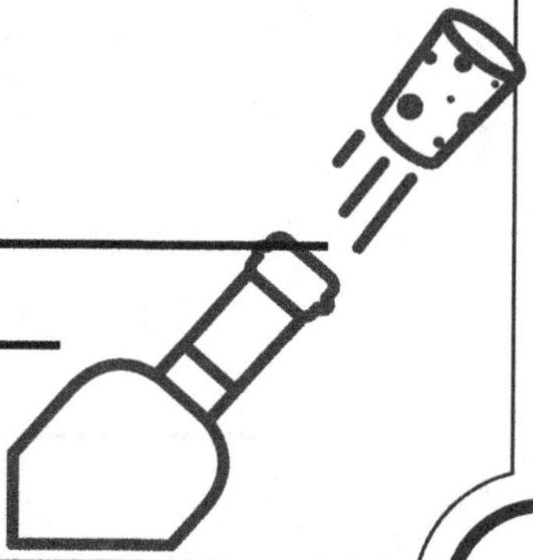

Color/Style: Red White Rose' Sparkling Effervescent Fortified
Appearance: Thin Thick
Dry/Sweet Spectrum: Dry 1 2 3 4 5 6 7 8 9 10 Sweet
Body: Light Light to Medium Medium Medium to Full Full Overall
Tasting Experience: Poor 1 2 3 4 5 6 7 8 9 10 Excellent

Comments:

____

____

____

____

Recommended Not Recommended

Circle One

Wine: ____________________ Date Tasted: __________

Region/Country: ____________________

Grape: ____________________

% Alcohol: ____________________

Producer: ____________ Vintage: ____________

Importer/Distributor: ____________

Price: ____________

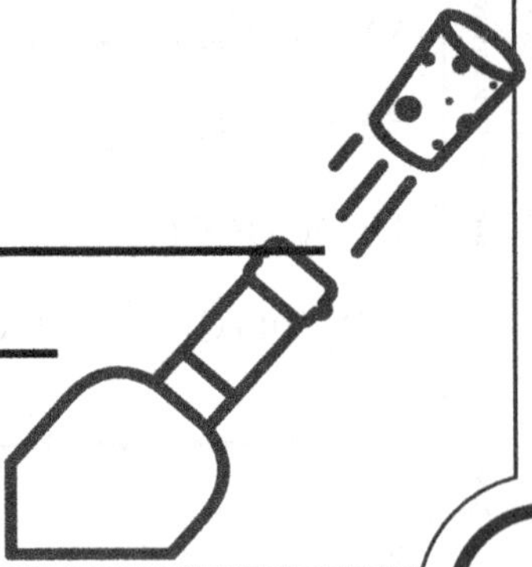

Color/Style: Red White Rose' Sparkling Effervescent Fortified

Appearance: Thin Thick

Dry/Sweet Spectrum: Dry 1 2 3 4 5 6 7 8 9 10 Sweet

Body: Light Light to Medium Medium Medium to Full Full Overall

Tasting Experience: Poor 1 2 3 4 5 6 7 8 9 10 Excellent

Comments:

Recommended Not Recommended

Circle One

Wine: ________________ Date Tasted: ________

Region/Country: ________________

Grape: ________________

% Alcohol: ________________

Producer: ____________ Vintage: ____________

Importer/Distributor: ____________

Price: ____________

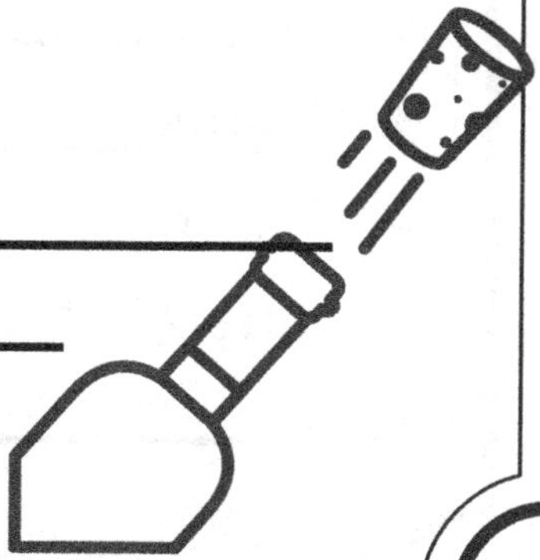

Color/Style: Red White Rose' Sparkling Effervescent Fortified

Appearance: Thin Thick

Dry/Sweet Spectrum: Dry 1 2 3 4 5 6 7 8 9 10 Sweet

Body: Light Light to Medium Medium Medium to Full Full Overall

Tasting Experience: Poor 1 2 3 4 5 6 7 8 9 10 Excellent

Comments:

____

____

____

____

Recommended Not Recommended

Circle One

Wine: ____________________ Date Tasted: __________

Region/Country: ____________________

Grape: ____________________

% Alcohol: ____________________

Producer: ____________ Vintage: ____________

Importer/Distributor: ____________

Price: ____________

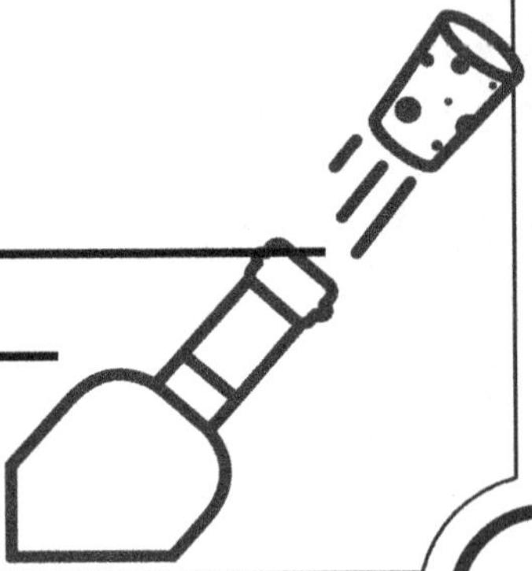

Color/Style: Red White Rose' Sparkling Effervescent Fortified

Appearance: Thin Thick

Dry/Sweet Spectrum: Dry 1 2 3 4 5 6 7 8 9 10 Sweet

Body: Light Light to Medium Medium Medium to Full Full Overall

Tasting Experience: Poor 1 2 3 4 5 6 7 8 9 10 Excellent

Comments:

Recommended Not Recommended

Circle One

Wine: ____________________ Date Tasted: __________

Region/Country: ____________________

Grape: ____________________

% Alcohol: ____________________

Producer: ____________ Vintage: ____________

Importer/Distributor: ____________

Price: ____________

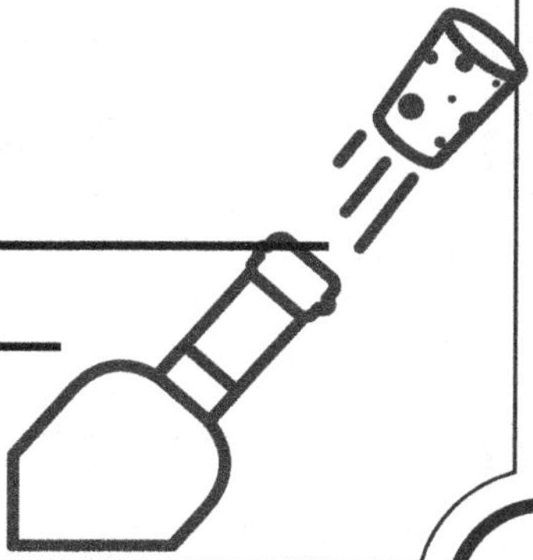

Color/Style: Red White Rose' Sparkling Effervescent Fortified

Appearance: Thin Thick

Dry/Sweet Spectrum: Dry 1 2 3 4 5 6 7 8 9 10 Sweet

Body: Light Light to Medium Medium Medium to Full Full Overall

Tasting Experience: Poor 1 2 3 4 5 6 7 8 9 10 Excellent

Comments:

Recommended Not Recommended

Circle One

Wine: ____________________ Date Tasted: __________

Region/Country: ____________________

Grape: ____________________

% Alcohol: ____________________

Producer: ____________ Vintage: ____________

Importer/Distributor: ____________

Price: ____________

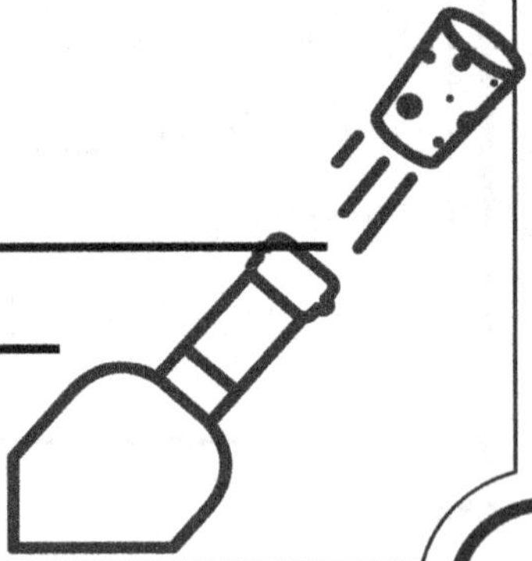

Color/Style: Red White Rose' Sparkling Effervescent Fortified

Appearance: Thin Thick

Dry/Sweet Spectrum: Dry 1 2 3 4 5 6 7 8 9 10 Sweet

Body: Light Light to Medium Medium Medium to Full Full Overall

Tasting Experience: Poor 1 2 3 4 5 6 7 8 9 10 Excellent

Comments:

Recommended Not Recommended

Circle One

Wine: ____________________ Date Tasted: __________

Region/Country: ____________________

Grape: ____________________

% Alcohol: ____________________

Producer: ____________ Vintage: ____________

Importer/Distributor: ____________

Price: ____________

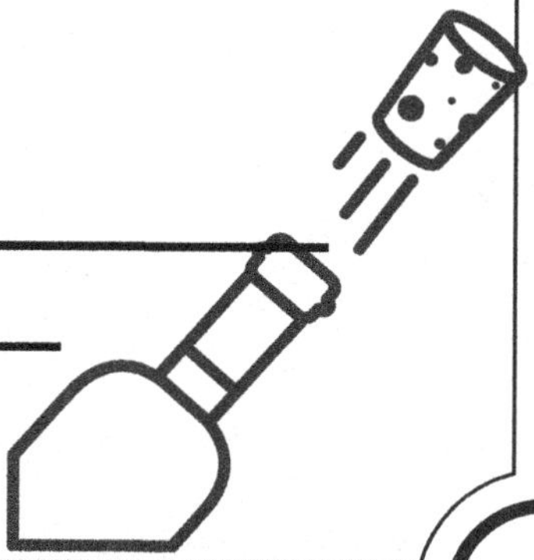

Color/Style: Red White Rose' Sparkling Effervescent Fortified

Appearance: Thin Thick

Dry/Sweet Spectrum: Dry 1 2 3 4 5 6 7 8 9 10 Sweet

Body: Light Light to Medium Medium Medium to Full Full Overall

Tasting Experience: Poor 1 2 3 4 5 6 7 8 9 10 Excellent

Comments:

____

____

____

____

Recommended Not Recommended

Circle One

Wine: ____________________ Date Tasted: __________

Region/Country: ____________________

Grape: ____________________

% Alcohol: ____________________

Producer: ____________ Vintage: ____________

Importer/Distributor: ____________

Price: ____________

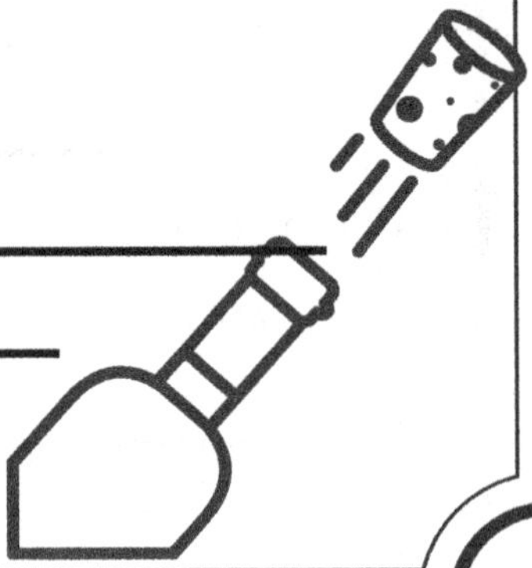

Color/Style: Red White Rose' Sparkling Effervescent Fortified

Appearance: Thin Thick

Dry/Sweet Spectrum: Dry 1 2 3 4 5 6 7 8 9 10 Sweet

Body: Light Light to Medium Medium Medium to Full Full Overall

Tasting Experience: Poor 1 2 3 4 5 6 7 8 9 10 Excellent

Comments:

Recommended Not Recommended

Circle One

Wine: ____________ Date Tasted: ________

Region/Country: ____________

Grape: ____________

% Alcohol: ____________

Producer: ________ Vintage: ________

Importer/Distributor: ________

Price: ________

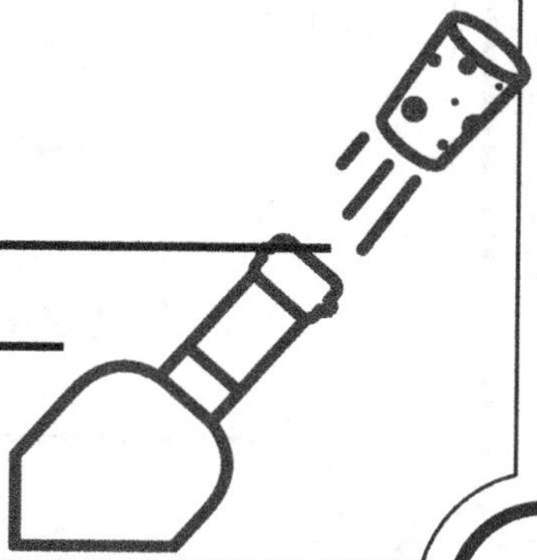

Color/Style: Red White Rose' Sparkling Effervescent Fortified

Appearance: Thin Thick

Dry/Sweet Spectrum: Dry 1 2 3 4 5 6 7 8 9 10 Sweet

Body: Light Light to Medium Medium Medium to Full Full Overall

Tasting Experience: Poor 1 2 3 4 5 6 7 8 9 10 Excellent

Comments:

____

____

____

____

Recommended Not Recommended

Circle One

Wine: ____________________ Date Tasted: ________

Region/Country: ____________________

Grape: ____________________

% Alcohol: ____________________

Producer: ____________ Vintage: ____________

Importer/Distributor: ____________

Price: ____________

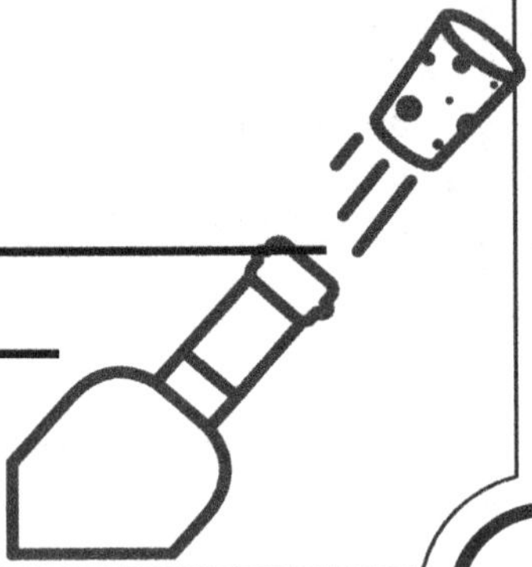

Color/Style: Red White Rose' Sparkling Effervescent Fortified
Appearance: Thin Thick
Dry/Sweet Spectrum: Dry 1 2 3 4 5 6 7 8 9 10 Sweet
Body: Light Light to Medium Medium Medium to Full Full Overall
Tasting Experience: Poor 1 2 3 4 5 6 7 8 9 10 Excellent

Comments:

____

____

____

____

Recommended Not Recommended

Circle One

Wine: ____________________ Date Tasted: ________

Region/Country: ____________________

Grape: ____________________

% Alcohol: ____________________

Producer: ____________ Vintage: ____________

Importer/Distributor: ____________

Price: ____________

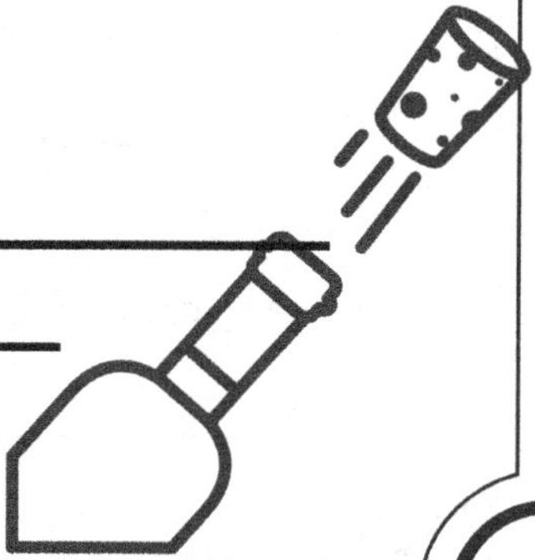

Color/Style: Red White Rose' Sparkling Effervescent Fortified

Appearance: Thin Thick

Dry/Sweet Spectrum: Dry 1 2 3 4 5 6 7 8 9 10 Sweet

Body: Light Light to Medium Medium Medium to Full Full Overall

Tasting Experience: Poor 1 2 3 4 5 6 7 8 9 10 Excellent

Comments:

____

____

____

____

Recommended Not Recommended

Circle One

Wine: ____________________ Date Tasted: __________

Region/Country: ____________________

Grape: ____________________

% Alcohol: ____________________

Producer: ____________ Vintage: ____________

Importer/Distributor: ____________

Price: ____________

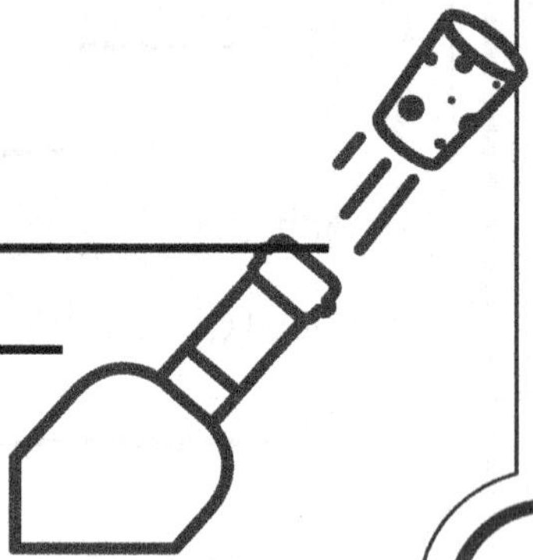

Color/Style: Red White Rose' Sparkling Effervescent Fortified

Appearance: Thin Thick

Dry/Sweet Spectrum: Dry 1 2 3 4 5 6 7 8 9 10 Sweet

Body: Light Light to Medium Medium Medium to Full Full Overall

Tasting Experience: Poor 1 2 3 4 5 6 7 8 9 10 Excellent

Comments:

____

____

____

____

Recommended Not Recommended

Circle One

Wine: ______________________ Date Tasted: __________

Region/Country: ______________________

Grape: ______________________

% Alcohol: ______________________

Producer: ______________ Vintage: ______________

Importer/Distributor: ______________

Price: ______________

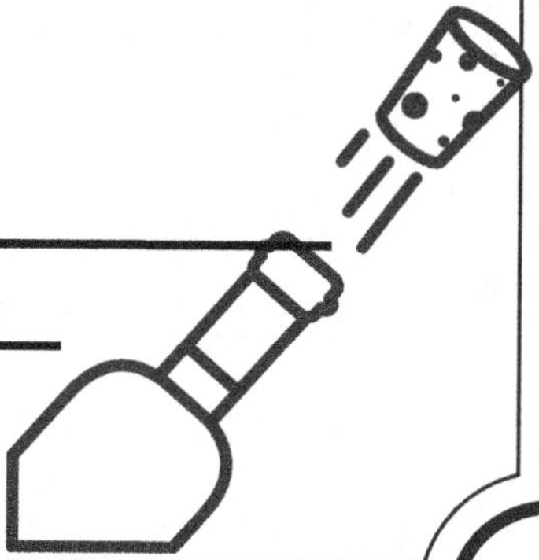

Color/Style: Red White Rose' Sparkling Effervescent Fortified

Appearance: Thin Thick

Dry/Sweet Spectrum: Dry 1 2 3 4 5 6 7 8 9 10 Sweet

Body: Light Light to Medium Medium Medium to Full Full Overall

Tasting Experience: Poor 1 2 3 4 5 6 7 8 9 10 Excellent

Comments:

____

____

____

____

Recommended Not Recommended

Circle One

Wine: ____________________ Date Tasted: __________

Region/Country: ____________________

Grape: ____________________

% Alcohol: ____________________

Producer: ____________ Vintage: ____________

Importer/Distributor: ____________

Price: ____________

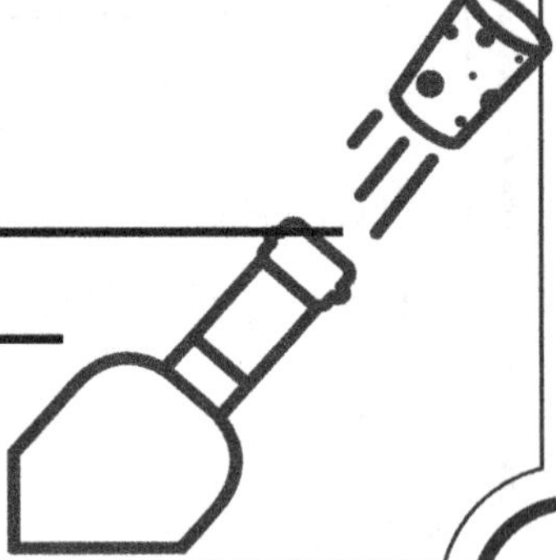

Color/Style: Red White Rose' Sparkling Effervescent Fortified

Appearance: Thin Thick

Dry/Sweet Spectrum: Dry 1 2 3 4 5 6 7 8 9 10 Sweet

Body: Light Light to Medium Medium Medium to Full Full Overall

Tasting Experience: Poor 1 2 3 4 5 6 7 8 9 10 Excellent

Comments:

Recommended Not Recommended

Circle One

Wine: ____________________ Date Tasted: __________

Region/Country: ____________________

Grape: ____________________

% Alcohol: ____________________

Producer: ____________ Vintage: ____________

Importer/Distributor: ____________

Price: ____________

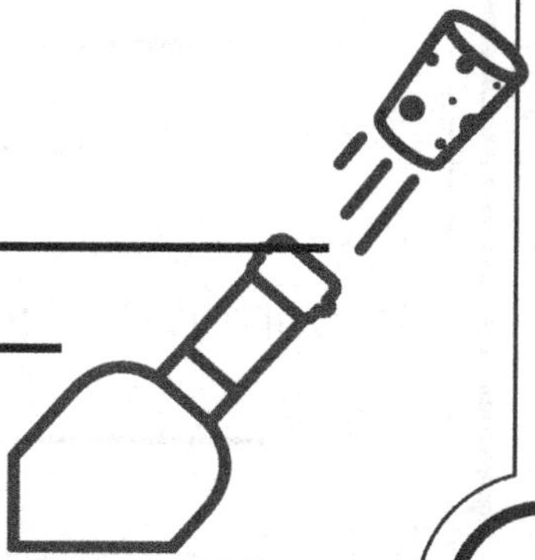

Color/Style: Red White Rose' Sparkling Effervescent Fortified

Appearance: Thin Thick

Dry/Sweet Spectrum: Dry 1 2 3 4 5 6 7 8 9 10 Sweet

Body: Light Light to Medium Medium Medium to Full Full Overall

Tasting Experience: Poor 1 2 3 4 5 6 7 8 9 10 Excellent

Comments:

____

____

____

____

Recommended Not Recommended

Circle One

Wine: ____________________ Date Tasted: __________

Region/Country: ____________________

Grape: ____________________

% Alcohol: ____________________

Producer: ____________ Vintage: ____________

Importer/Distributor: ____________

Price: ____________

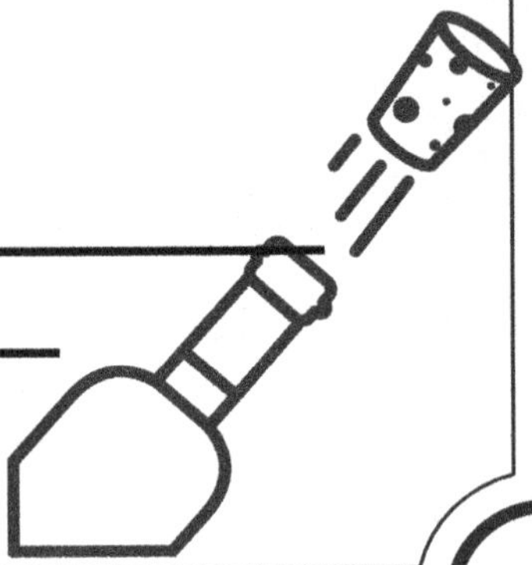

Color/Style: Red White Rose' Sparkling Effervescent Fortified

Appearance: Thin Thick

Dry/Sweet Spectrum: Dry 1 2 3 4 5 6 7 8 9 10 Sweet

Body: Light Light to Medium Medium Medium to Full Full Overall

Tasting Experience: Poor 1 2 3 4 5 6 7 8 9 10 Excellent

Comments:

Recommended Not Recommended

Circle One

Wine: ________________ Date Tasted: ________

Region/Country: ________________

Grape: ________________

% Alcohol: ________________

Producer: __________ Vintage: __________

Importer/Distributor: __________

Price: __________

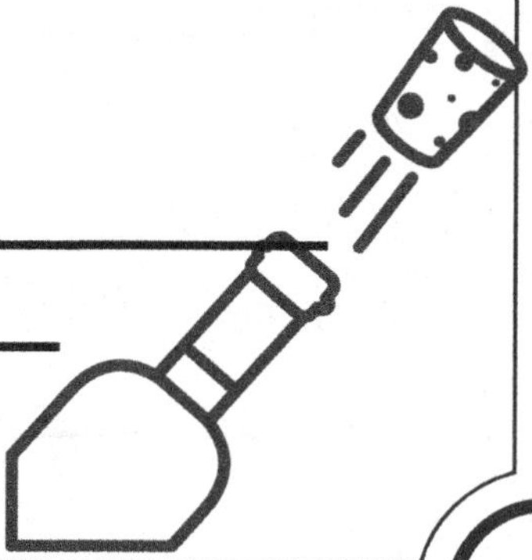

Color/Style: Red White Rose' Sparkling Effervescent Fortified

Appearance: Thin Thick

Dry/Sweet Spectrum: Dry 1 2 3 4 5 6 7 8 9 10 Sweet

Body: Light Light to Medium Medium Medium to Full Full Overall

Tasting Experience: Poor 1 2 3 4 5 6 7 8 9 10 Excellent

Comments:

____

____

____

____

Recommended Not Recommended

Circle One

Wine: ______________________ Date Tasted: __________

Region/Country: ______________________

Grape: ______________________

% Alcohol: ______________________

Producer: ____________ Vintage: ____________

Importer/Distributor: ______________

Price: ______________

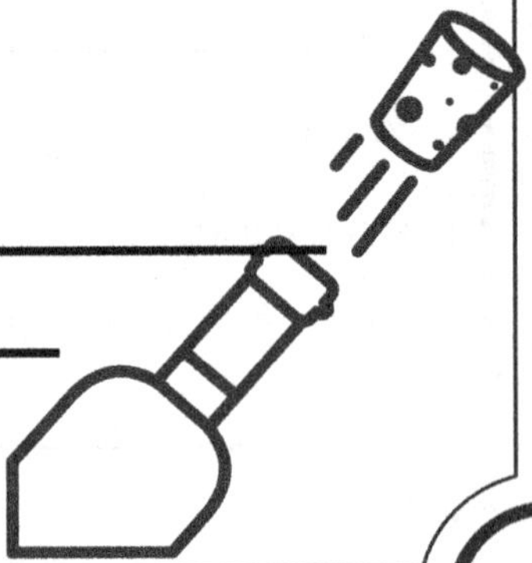

Color/Style: Red White Rose' Sparkling Effervescent Fortified

Appearance: Thin Thick

Dry/Sweet Spectrum: Dry 1 2 3 4 5 6 7 8 9 10 Sweet

Body: Light Light to Medium Medium Medium to Full Full Overall

Tasting Experience: Poor 1 2 3 4 5 6 7 8 9 10 Excellent

Comments:

Recommended Not Recommended

Circle One

Wine: ______________________ Date Tasted: __________

Region/Country: ______________________

Grape: ______________________

% Alcohol: ______________________

Producer: ______________ Vintage: ______________

Importer/Distributor: ______________

Price: ______________

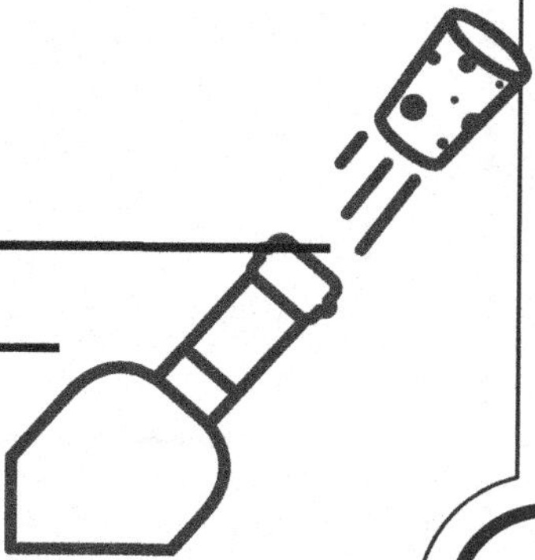

Color/Style: Red White Rose' Sparkling Effervescent Fortified

Appearance: Thin Thick

Dry/Sweet Spectrum: Dry 1 2 3 4 5 6 7 8 9 10 Sweet

Body: Light Light to Medium Medium Medium to Full Full Overall

Tasting Experience: Poor 1 2 3 4 5 6 7 8 9 10 Excellent

Comments:

____

____

____

____

Recommended Not Recommended

Circle One

Wine: ____________________ Date Tasted: __________

Region/Country: ____________________

Grape: ____________________

% Alcohol: ____________________

Producer: ____________ Vintage: ____________

Importer/Distributor: ____________

Price: ____________

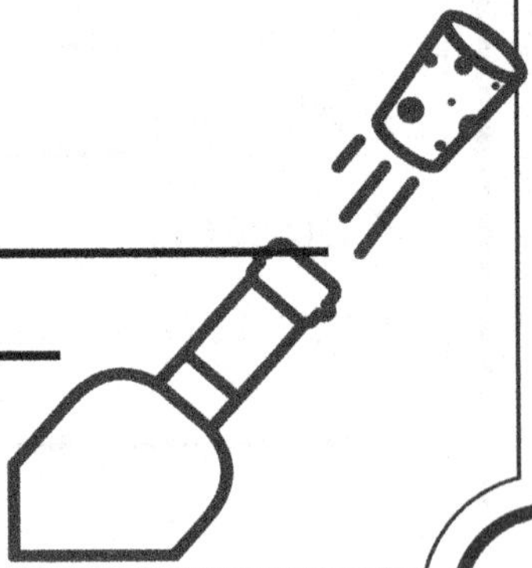

Color/Style: Red White Rose' Sparkling Effervescent Fortified

Appearance: Thin Thick

Dry/Sweet Spectrum: Dry 1 2 3 4 5 6 7 8 9 10 Sweet

Body: Light Light to Medium Medium Medium to Full Full Overall

Tasting Experience: Poor 1 2 3 4 5 6 7 8 9 10 Excellent

Comments:

Recommended Not Recommended

Circle One

Wine: ______________ Date Tasted: ________

Region/Country: ______________

Grape: ______________

% Alcohol: ______________

Producer: __________ Vintage: __________

Importer/Distributor: __________

Price: __________

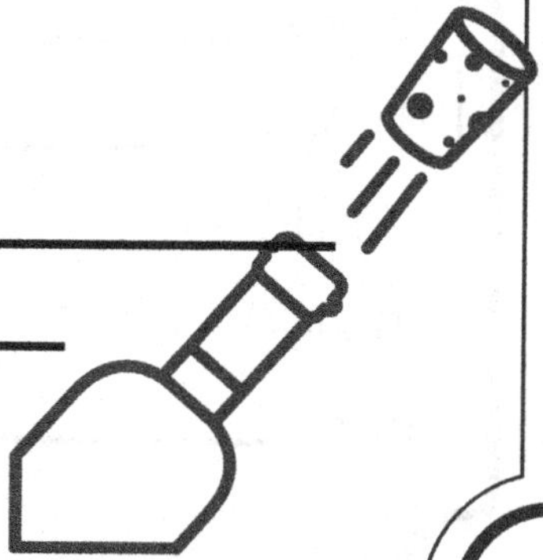

Color/Style: Red White Rose' Sparkling Effervescent Fortified

Appearance: Thin Thick

Dry/Sweet Spectrum: Dry 1 2 3 4 5 6 7 8 9 10 Sweet

Body: Light Light to Medium Medium Medium to Full Full Overall

Tasting Experience: Poor 1 2 3 4 5 6 7 8 9 10 Excellent

Comments:

Recommended Not Recommended

Circle One

Wine: ____________ Date Tasted: ________

Region/Country: ____________

Grape: ____________

% Alcohol: ____________

Producer: ________ Vintage: ________

Importer/Distributor: ________

Price: ________

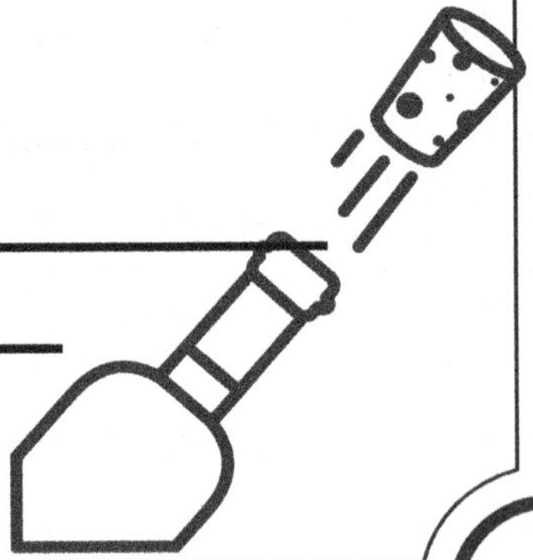

Color/Style: Red White Rose' Sparkling Effervescent Fortified

Appearance: Thin Thick

Dry/Sweet Spectrum: Dry 1 2 3 4 5 6 7 8 9 10 Sweet

Body: Light Light to Medium Medium Medium to Full Full Overall

Tasting Experience: Poor 1 2 3 4 5 6 7 8 9 10 Excellent

Comments:

Recommended Not Recommended

Circle One

Wine: ____________ Date Tasted: ________

Region/Country: ____________

Grape: ____________

% Alcohol: ____________

Producer: ________ Vintage: ________

Importer/Distributor: ________

Price: ________

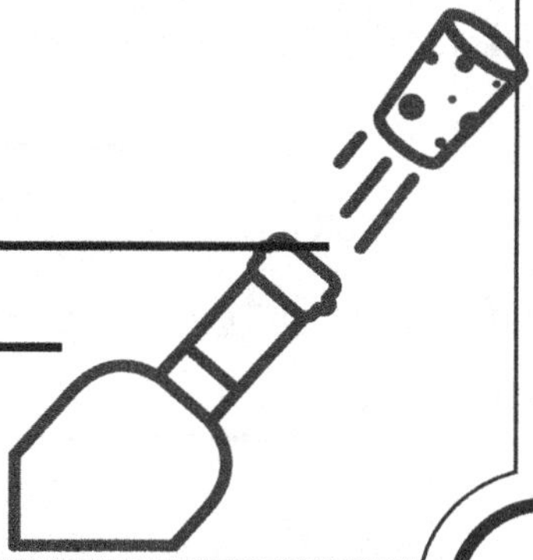

Color/Style: Red White Rose' Sparkling Effervescent Fortified

Appearance: Thin Thick

Dry/Sweet Spectrum: Dry 1 2 3 4 5 6 7 8 9 10 Sweet

Body: Light Light to Medium Medium Medium to Full Full Overall

Tasting Experience: Poor 1 2 3 4 5 6 7 8 9 10 Excellent

Comments:

____

____

____

____

Recommended Not Recommended

Circle One

Wine: ____________________ Date Tasted: __________

Region/Country: ____________________

Grape: ____________________

% Alcohol: ____________________

Producer: ____________ Vintage: ____________

Importer/Distributor: ____________

Price: ____________

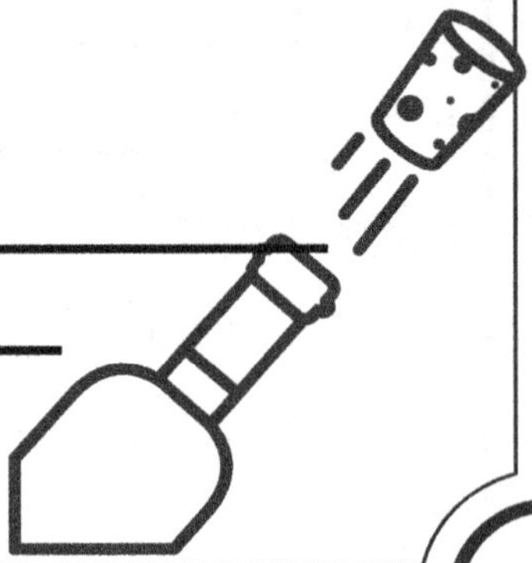

Color/Style: Red White Rose' Sparkling Effervescent Fortified

Appearance: Thin Thick

Dry/Sweet Spectrum: Dry 1 2 3 4 5 6 7 8 9 10 Sweet

Body: Light Light to Medium Medium Medium to Full Full Overall

Tasting Experience: Poor 1 2 3 4 5 6 7 8 9 10 Excellent

Comments:

____

____

____

____

Recommended Not Recommended

Circle One

Wine: ____________ Date Tasted: ________

Region/Country: ____________

Grape: ____________

% Alcohol: ____________

Producer: ________ Vintage: ________

Importer/Distributor: ________

Price: ________

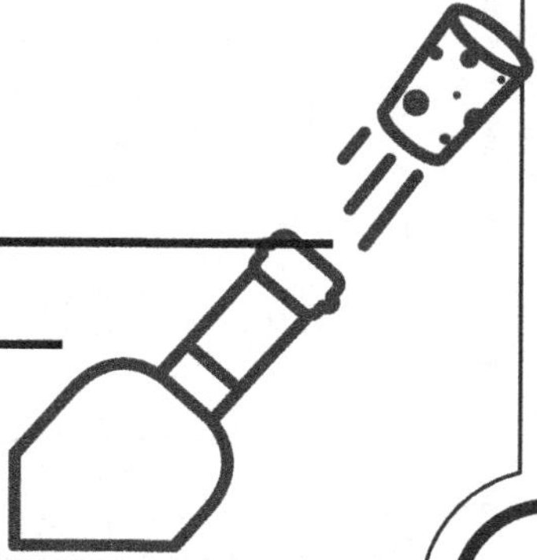

Color/Style: Red White Rose' Sparkling Effervescent Fortified

Appearance: Thin Thick

Dry/Sweet Spectrum: Dry 1 2 3 4 5 6 7 8 9 10 Sweet

Body: Light Light to Medium Medium Medium to Full Full Overall

Tasting Experience: Poor 1 2 3 4 5 6 7 8 9 10 Excellent

Comments:

Recommended Not Recommended

Circle One

Wine: ____________________ Date Tasted: _________

Region/Country: ____________________

Grape: ____________________

% Alcohol: ____________________

Producer: ____________ Vintage: ____________

Importer/Distributor: ____________

Price: ____________

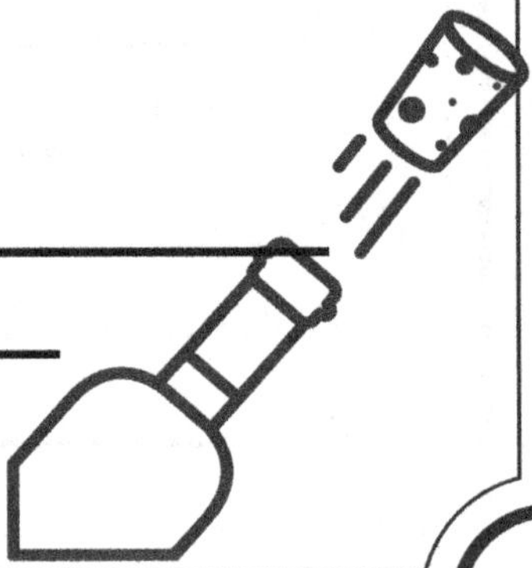

Color/Style: Red White Rose' Sparkling Effervescent Fortified

Appearance: Thin Thick

Dry/Sweet Spectrum: Dry 1 2 3 4 5 6 7 8 9 10 Sweet

Body: Light Light to Medium Medium Medium to Full Full Overall

Tasting Experience: Poor 1 2 3 4 5 6 7 8 9 10 Excellent

Comments:

Recommended Not Recommended

Circle One

Wine: ______________________ Date Tasted: __________

Region/Country: ______________________

Grape: ______________________

% Alcohol: ______________________

Producer: ______________ Vintage: ______________

Importer/Distributor: ______________

Price: ______________

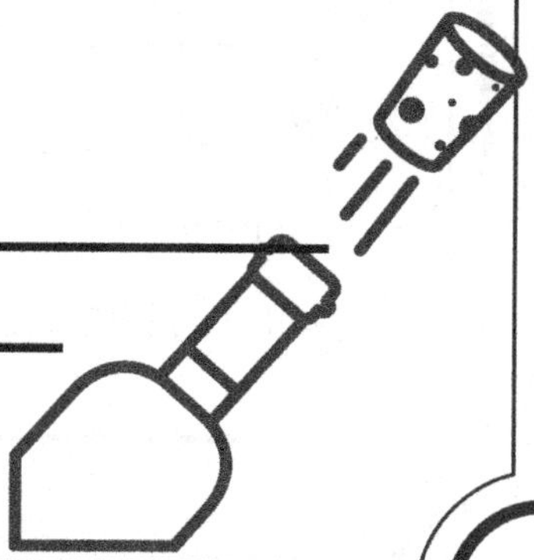

Color/Style: Red White Rose' Sparkling Effervescent Fortified

Appearance: Thin Thick

Dry/Sweet Spectrum: Dry 1 2 3 4 5 6 7 8 9 10 Sweet

Body: Light Light to Medium Medium Medium to Full Full Overall

Tasting Experience: Poor 1 2 3 4 5 6 7 8 9 10 Excellent

Comments:

Recommended Not Recommended

Circle One

Wine: ____________________ Date Tasted: __________

Region/Country: ____________________

Grape: ____________________

% Alcohol: ____________________

Producer: ____________ Vintage: ____________

Importer/Distributor: ____________

Price: ____________

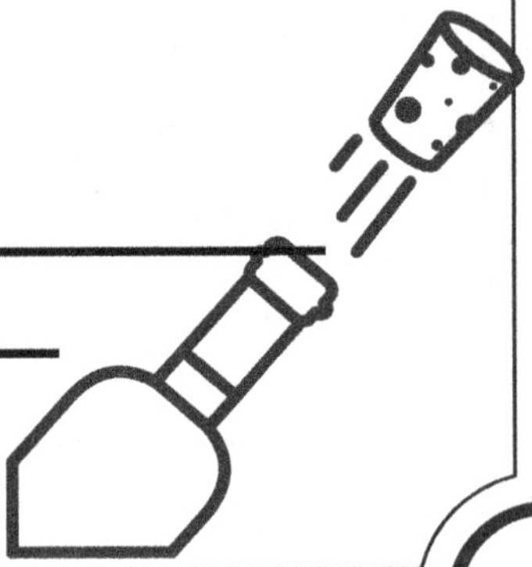

Color/Style: Red White Rose' Sparkling Effervescent Fortified

Appearance: Thin Thick

Dry/Sweet Spectrum: Dry 1 2 3 4 5 6 7 8 9 10 Sweet

Body: Light Light to Medium Medium Medium to Full Full Overall

Tasting Experience: Poor 1 2 3 4 5 6 7 8 9 10 Excellent

Comments:

____

____

____

____

Recommended Not Recommended

Circle One

Wine: ____________________ Date Tasted: __________

Region/Country: ____________________

Grape: ____________________

% Alcohol: ____________________

Producer: ____________ Vintage: ____________

Importer/Distributor: ____________

Price: ____________

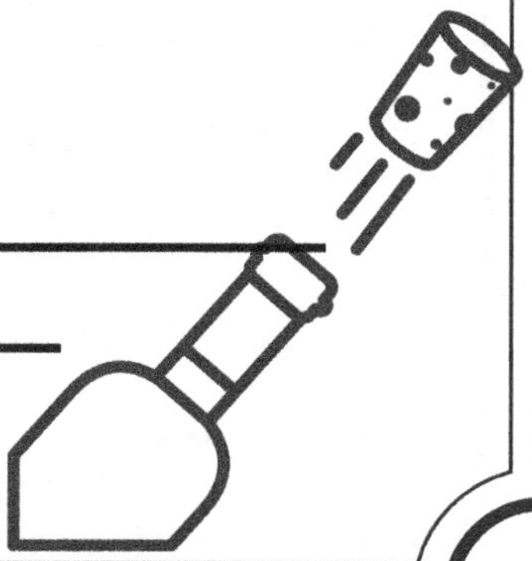

Color/Style: Red White Rose' Sparkling Effervescent Fortified

Appearance: Thin Thick

Dry/Sweet Spectrum: Dry 1 2 3 4 5 6 7 8 9 10 Sweet

Body: Light Light to Medium Medium Medium to Full Full Overall

Tasting Experience: Poor 1 2 3 4 5 6 7 8 9 10 Excellent

Comments:

____

____

____

____

Recommended Not Recommended

Circle One

Wine: ____________________ Date Tasted: ________

Region/Country: ____________________

Grape: ____________________

% Alcohol: ____________________

Producer: ____________ Vintage: ____________

Importer/Distributor: ____________

Price: ____________

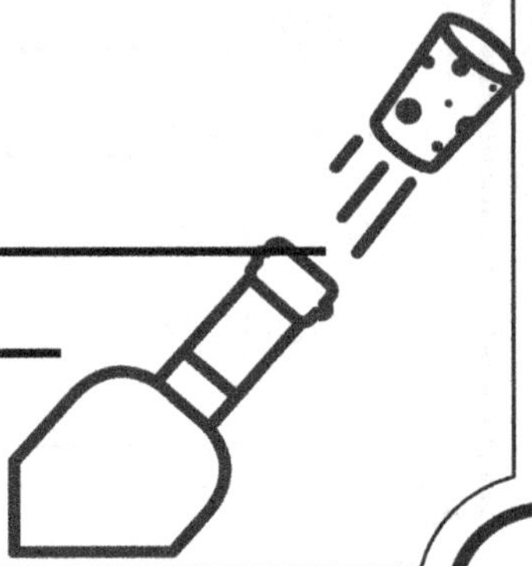

Color/Style: Red White Rose' Sparkling Effervescent Fortified

Appearance: Thin Thick

Dry/Sweet Spectrum: Dry 1 2 3 4 5 6 7 8 9 10 Sweet

Body: Light Light to Medium Medium Medium to Full Full Overall

Tasting Experience: Poor 1 2 3 4 5 6 7 8 9 10 Excellent

Comments:

____

____

____

____

Recommended Not Recommended

Circle One

Wine: ____________ Date Tasted: ________

Region/Country: ____________

Grape: ____________

% Alcohol: ____________

Producer: ________ Vintage: ________

Importer/Distributor: ________

Price: ________

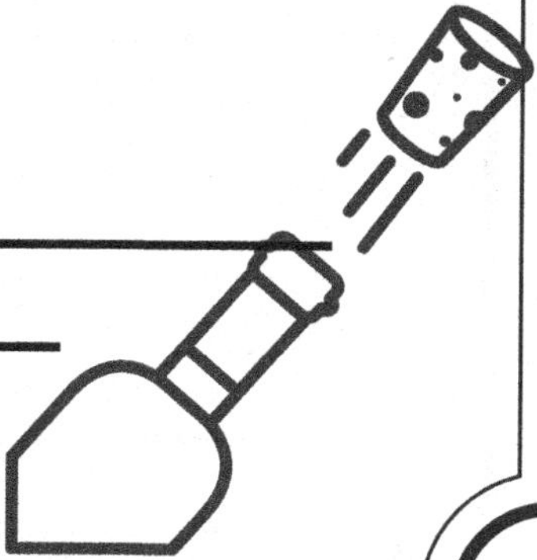

Color/Style: Red White Rose' Sparkling Effervescent Fortified

Appearance: Thin Thick

Dry/Sweet Spectrum: Dry 1 2 3 4 5 6 7 8 9 10 Sweet

Body: Light Light to Medium Medium Medium to Full Full Overall

Tasting Experience: Poor 1 2 3 4 5 6 7 8 9 10 Excellent

Comments:

____

____

____

____

Recommended Not Recommended

Circle One

Wine: ______________________ Date Tasted: __________

Region/Country: ______________________

Grape: ______________________

% Alcohol: ______________________

Producer: ______________ Vintage: ______________

Importer/Distributor: ______________

Price: ______________

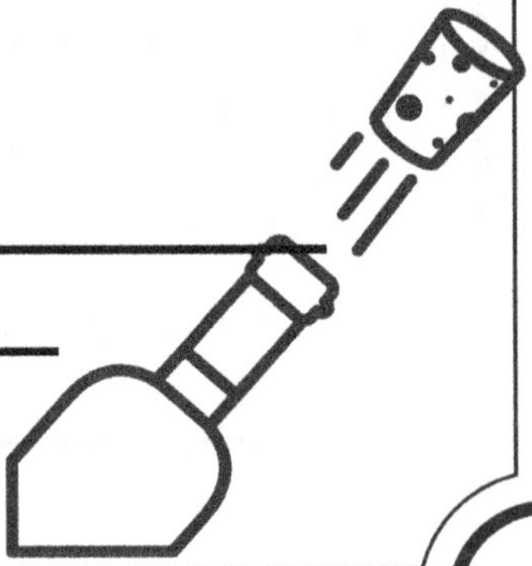

Color/Style: Red White Rose' Sparkling Effervescent Fortified

Appearance: Thin Thick

Dry/Sweet Spectrum: Dry 1 2 3 4 5 6 7 8 9 10 Sweet

Body: Light Light to Medium Medium Medium to Full Full Overall

Tasting Experience: Poor 1 2 3 4 5 6 7 8 9 10 Excellent

Comments:

Recommended Not Recommended

Circle One

Wine: ______________ Date Tasted: ________

Region/Country: ______________

Grape: ______________

% Alcohol: ______________

Producer: __________ Vintage: __________

Importer/Distributor: __________

Price: __________

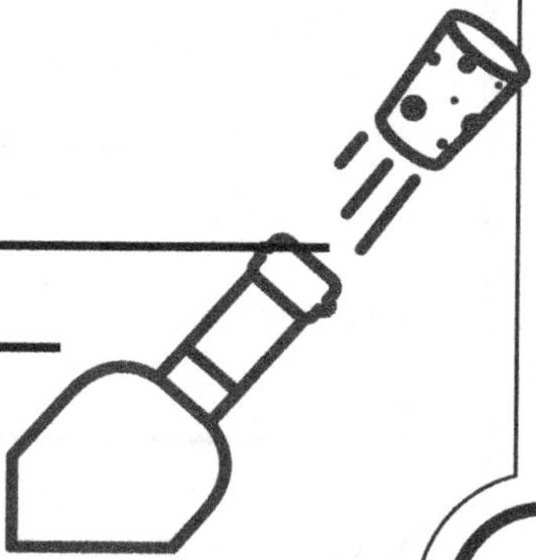

Color/Style: Red White Rose' Sparkling Effervescent Fortified

Appearance: Thin Thick

Dry/Sweet Spectrum: Dry 1 2 3 4 5 6 7 8 9 10 Sweet

Body: Light Light to Medium Medium Medium to Full Full Overall

Tasting Experience: Poor 1 2 3 4 5 6 7 8 9 10 Excellent

Comments:

____

____

____

____

Recommended Not Recommended

Circle One

Wine: ____________________ Date Tasted: __________

Region/Country: ____________________

Grape: ____________________

% Alcohol: ____________________

Producer: ____________ Vintage: ____________

Importer/Distributor: ____________

Price: ____________

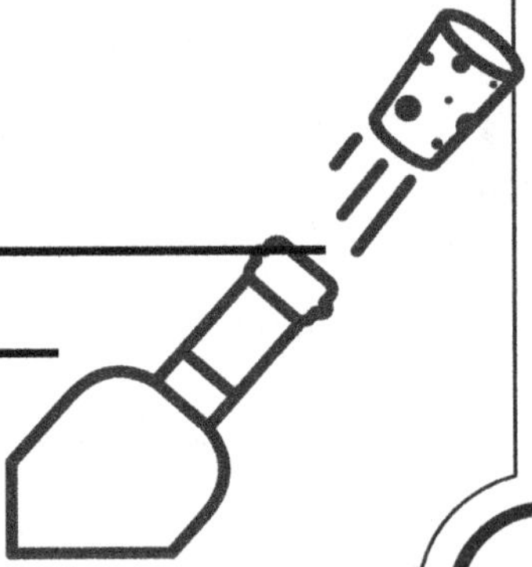

Color/Style: Red White Rose' Sparkling Effervescent Fortified
Appearance: Thin Thick
Dry/Sweet Spectrum: Dry 1 2 3 4 5 6 7 8 9 10 Sweet
Body: Light Light to Medium Medium Medium to Full Full Overall
Tasting Experience: Poor 1 2 3 4 5 6 7 8 9 10 Excellent

Comments:

Recommended Not Recommended

Circle One

Wine: ____________________ Date Tasted: ________

Region/Country: ____________________

Grape: ____________________

% Alcohol: ____________________

Producer: ____________ Vintage: ____________

Importer/Distributor: ____________

Price: ____________

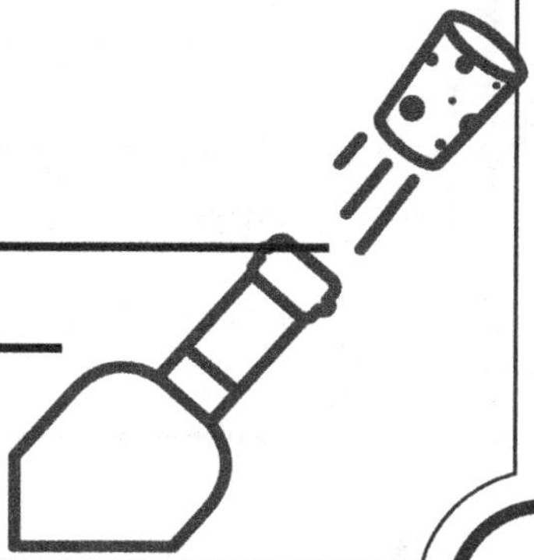

Color/Style: Red White Rose' Sparkling Effervescent Fortified

Appearance: Thin Thick

Dry/Sweet Spectrum: Dry 1 2 3 4 5 6 7 8 9 10 Sweet

Body: Light Light to Medium Medium Medium to Full Full Overall

Tasting Experience: Poor 1 2 3 4 5 6 7 8 9 10 Excellent

Comments:

____

____

____

____

Recommended Not Recommended

Circle One

Wine: ____________________ Date Tasted: ________

Region/Country: ____________________

Grape: ____________________

% Alcohol: ____________________

Producer: ____________ Vintage: ____________

Importer/Distributor: ____________

Price: ____________

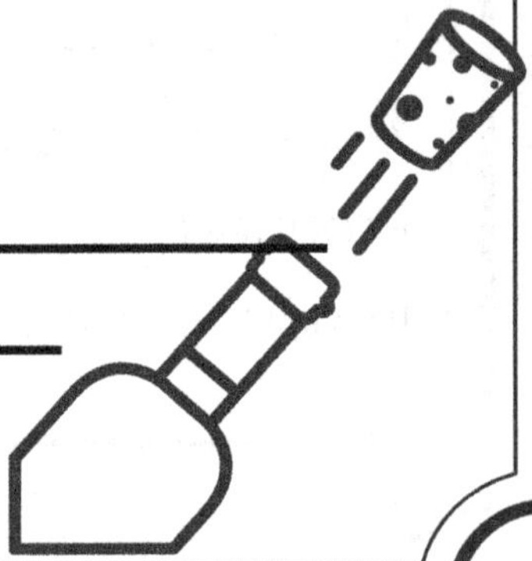

Color/Style: Red White Rose' Sparkling Effervescent Fortified

Appearance: Thin Thick

Dry/Sweet Spectrum: Dry 1 2 3 4 5 6 7 8 9 10 Sweet

Body: Light Light to Medium Medium Medium to Full Full Overall

Tasting Experience: Poor 1 2 3 4 5 6 7 8 9 10 Excellent

Comments:

Recommended Not Recommended

Circle One

Wine: ____________________ Date Tasted: ________

Region/Country: ____________________

Grape: ____________________

% Alcohol: ____________________

Producer: ____________ Vintage: ____________

Importer/Distributor: ____________

Price: ____________

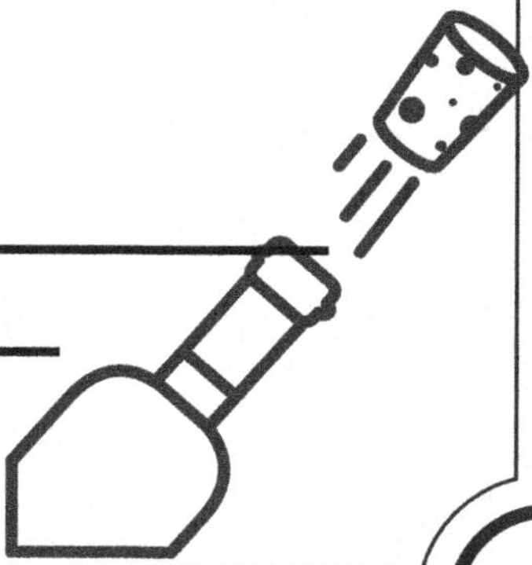

Color/Style: Red White Rose' Sparkling Effervescent Fortified

Appearance: Thin Thick

Dry/Sweet Spectrum: Dry 1 2 3 4 5 6 7 8 9 10 Sweet

Body: Light Light to Medium Medium Medium to Full Full Overall

Tasting Experience: Poor 1 2 3 4 5 6 7 8 9 10 Excellent

Comments:

____

____

____

____

Recommended Not Recommended

Circle One

Wine: ______________ Date Tasted: ________

Region/Country: ______________

Grape: ______________

% Alcohol: ______________

Producer: __________ Vintage: __________

Importer/Distributor: __________

Price: __________

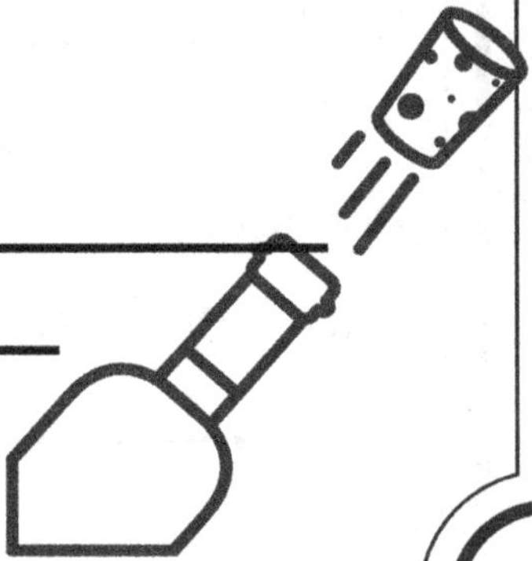

Color/Style: Red White Rose' Sparkling Effervescent Fortified

Appearance: Thin Thick

Dry/Sweet Spectrum: Dry 1 2 3 4 5 6 7 8 9 10 Sweet

Body: Light Light to Medium Medium Medium to Full Full Overall

Tasting Experience: Poor 1 2 3 4 5 6 7 8 9 10 Excellent

Comments:

____

____

____

____

Recommended Not Recommended

Circle One

Wine: ______________________ Date Tasted: __________

Region/Country: ______________________

Grape: ______________________

% Alcohol: ______________________

Producer: ______________ Vintage: ______________

Importer/Distributor: ______________

Price: ______________

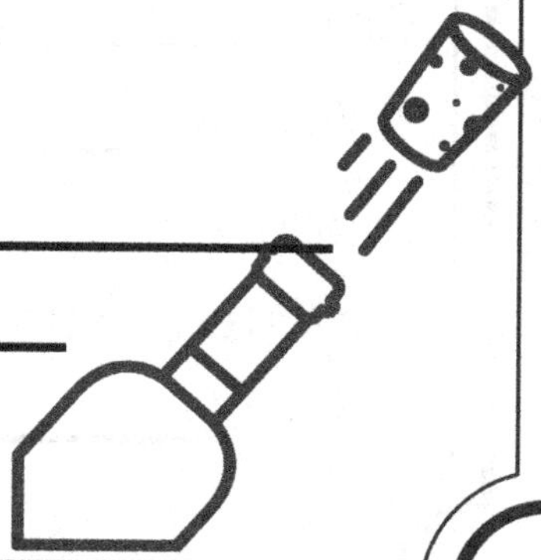

Color/Style: Red White Rose' Sparkling Effervescent Fortified

Appearance: Thin Thick

Dry/Sweet Spectrum: Dry 1 2 3 4 5 6 7 8 9 10 Sweet

Body: Light Light to Medium Medium Medium to Full Full Overall

Tasting Experience: Poor 1 2 3 4 5 6 7 8 9 10 Excellent

Comments:

____

____

____

____

Recommended Not Recommended

Circle One

Wine: ______________________ Date Tasted: __________

Region/Country: ______________________

Grape: ______________________

% Alcohol: ______________________

Producer: ____________ Vintage: ____________

Importer/Distributor: ____________

Price: ____________

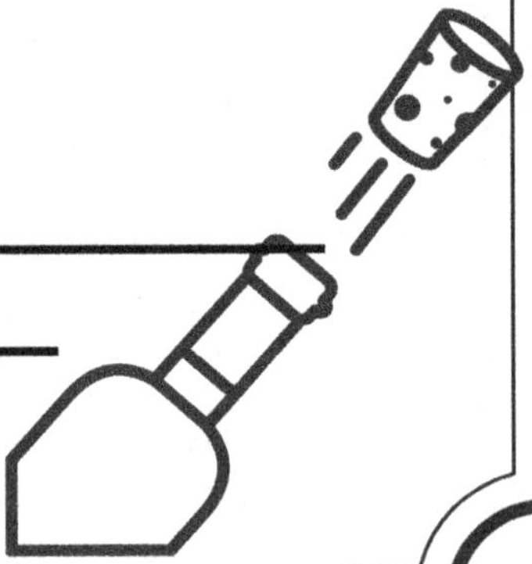

Color/Style: Red White Rose' Sparkling Effervescent Fortified

Appearance: Thin Thick

Dry/Sweet Spectrum: Dry 1 2 3 4 5 6 7 8 9 10 Sweet

Body: Light Light to Medium Medium Medium to Full Full Overall

Tasting Experience: Poor 1 2 3 4 5 6 7 8 9 10 Excellent

Comments:

____

____

____

____

Recommended Not Recommended

Circle One

Wine: ____________________ Date Tasted: ________

Region/Country: ____________________

Grape: ____________________

% Alcohol: ____________________

Producer: ____________ Vintage: ____________

Importer/Distributor: ____________

Price: ____________

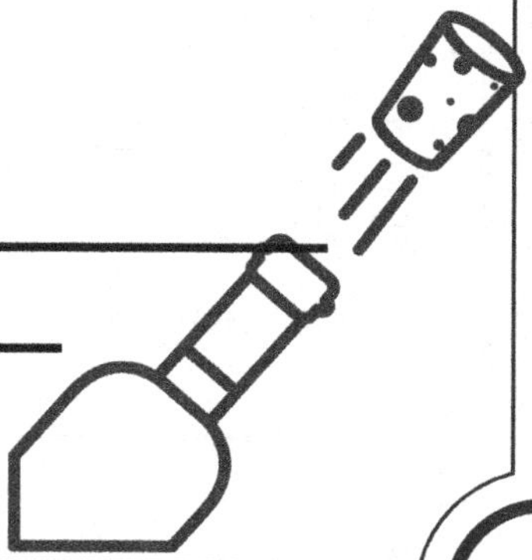

Color/Style: Red White Rose' Sparkling Effervescent Fortified

Appearance: Thin Thick

Dry/Sweet Spectrum: Dry 1 2 3 4 5 6 7 8 9 10 Sweet

Body: Light Light to Medium Medium Medium to Full Full Overall

Tasting Experience: Poor 1 2 3 4 5 6 7 8 9 10 Excellent

Comments:

____

____

____

____

Recommended Not Recommended

Circle One

Wine: ____________________ Date Tasted: ________

Region/Country: ____________________

Grape: ____________________

% Alcohol: ____________________

Producer: ____________ Vintage: ____________

Importer/Distributor: ____________

Price: ____________

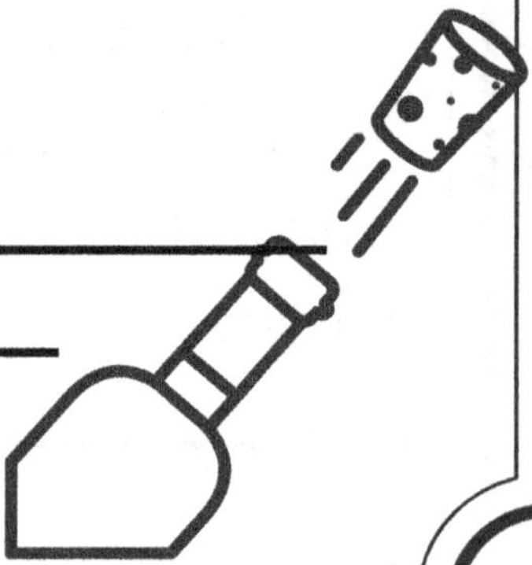

Color/Style: Red White Rose' Sparkling Effervescent Fortified

Appearance: Thin Thick

Dry/Sweet Spectrum: Dry 1 2 3 4 5 6 7 8 9 10 Sweet

Body: Light Light to Medium Medium Medium to Full Full Overall

Tasting Experience: Poor 1 2 3 4 5 6 7 8 9 10 Excellent

Comments:

Recommended Not Recommended

Circle One

Wine: ______________ Date Tasted: ________

Region/Country: ______________

Grape: ______________

% Alcohol: ______________

Producer: __________ Vintage: __________

Importer/Distributor: __________

Price: __________

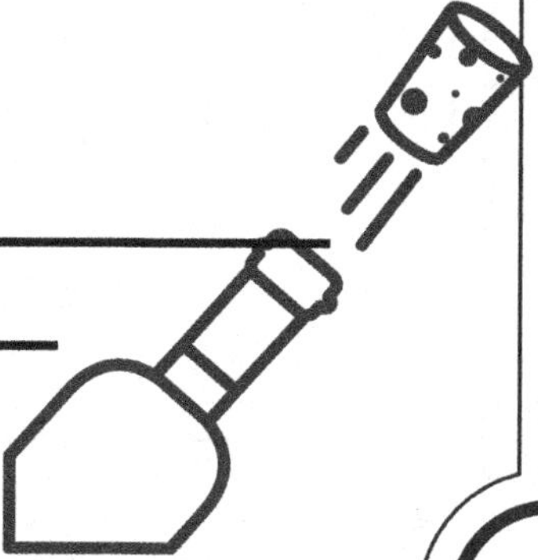

Color/Style: Red White Rose' Sparkling Effervescent Fortified

Appearance: Thin Thick

Dry/Sweet Spectrum: Dry 1 2 3 4 5 6 7 8 9 10 Sweet

Body: Light Light to Medium Medium Medium to Full Full Overall

Tasting Experience: Poor 1 2 3 4 5 6 7 8 9 10 Excellent

Comments:

____

____

____

____

Recommended Not Recommended

Circle One

Wine: ____________________ Date Tasted: __________

Region/Country: ____________________

Grape: ____________________

% Alcohol: ____________________

Producer: ____________ Vintage: ____________

Importer/Distributor: ____________

Price: ____________

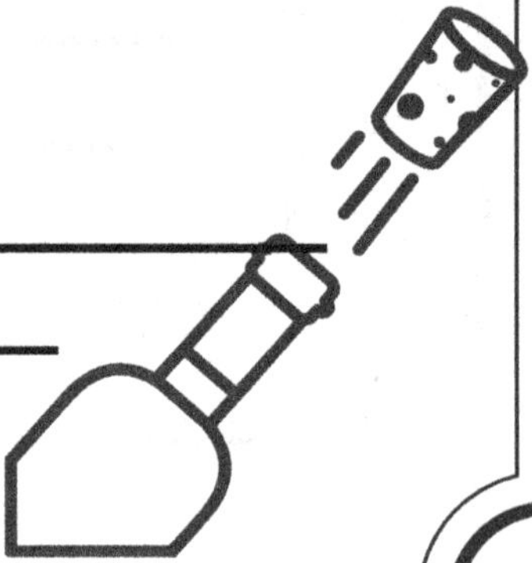

Color/Style: Red White Rose' Sparkling Effervescent Fortified

Appearance: Thin Thick

Dry/Sweet Spectrum: Dry 1 2 3 4 5 6 7 8 9 10 Sweet

Body: Light Light to Medium Medium Medium to Full Full Overall

Tasting Experience: Poor 1 2 3 4 5 6 7 8 9 10 Excellent

Comments:

____

____

____

____

Recommended Not Recommended

Circle One

Wine: ____________________ Date Tasted: __________

Region/Country: ____________________

Grape: ____________________

% Alcohol: ____________________

Producer: ____________ Vintage: ____________

Importer/Distributor: ____________

Price: ____________

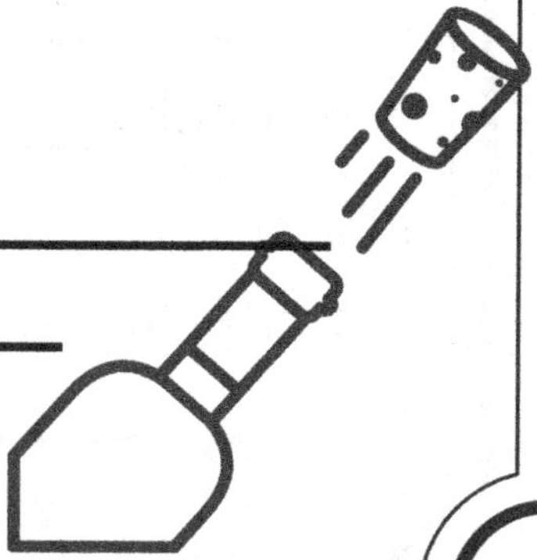

Color/Style: Red White Rose' Sparkling Effervescent Fortified

Appearance: Thin Thick

Dry/Sweet Spectrum: Dry 1 2 3 4 5 6 7 8 9 10 Sweet

Body: Light Light to Medium Medium Medium to Full Full Overall

Tasting Experience: Poor 1 2 3 4 5 6 7 8 9 10 Excellent

Comments:

____

____

____

____

Recommended Not Recommended

Circle One

Wine: ______________________ Date Tasted: ________

Region/Country: ______________________

Grape: ______________________

% Alcohol: ______________________

Producer: ______________ Vintage: ______________

Importer/Distributor: ______________

Price: ______________

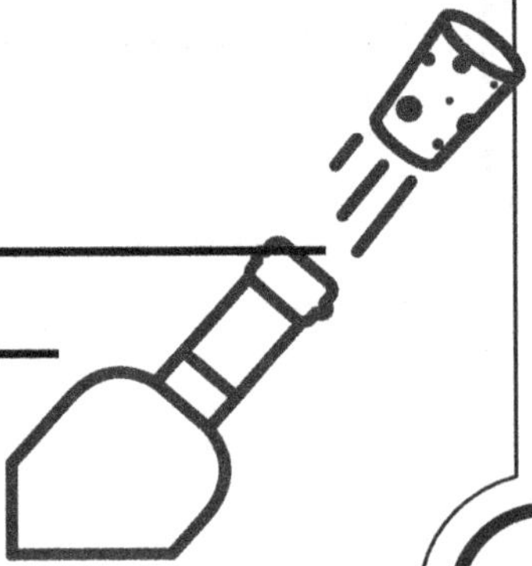

Color/Style: Red White Rose' Sparkling Effervescent Fortified

Appearance: Thin Thick

Dry/Sweet Spectrum: Dry 1 2 3 4 5 6 7 8 9 10 Sweet

Body: Light Light to Medium Medium Medium to Full Full Overall

Tasting Experience: Poor 1 2 3 4 5 6 7 8 9 10 Excellent

Comments:

____

____

____

____

Recommended Not Recommended

Circle One

Wine: ______________________ Date Tasted: __________

Region/Country: ______________________

Grape: ______________________

% Alcohol: ______________________

Producer: ______________ Vintage: ______________

Importer/Distributor: ______________

Price: ______________

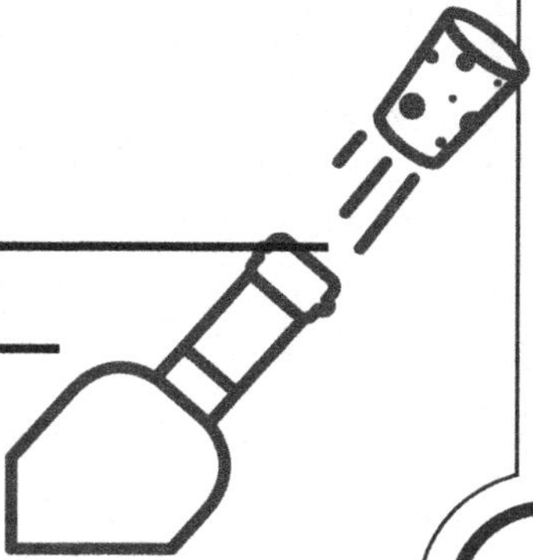

Color/Style: Red White Rose' Sparkling Effervescent Fortified

Appearance: Thin Thick

Dry/Sweet Spectrum: Dry 1 2 3 4 5 6 7 8 9 10 Sweet

Body: Light Light to Medium Medium Medium to Full Full Overall

Tasting Experience: Poor 1 2 3 4 5 6 7 8 9 10 Excellent

Comments:

____

____

____

____

Recommended Not Recommended

Circle One

Wine: ____________________ Date Tasted: __________

Region/Country: ____________________

Grape: ____________________

% Alcohol: ____________________

Producer: ____________ Vintage: ____________

Importer/Distributor: ____________

Price: ____________

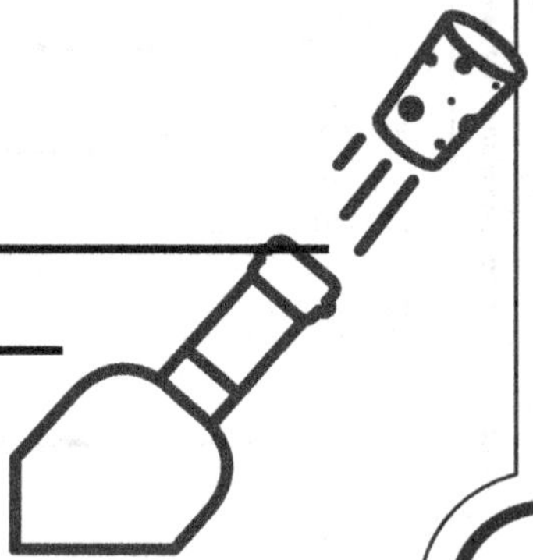

Color/Style: Red White Rose' Sparkling Effervescent Fortified

Appearance: Thin Thick

Dry/Sweet Spectrum: Dry 1 2 3 4 5 6 7 8 9 10 Sweet

Body: Light Light to Medium Medium Medium to Full Full Overall

Tasting Experience: Poor 1 2 3 4 5 6 7 8 9 10 Excellent

Comments:

Recommended Not Recommended

Circle One

Wine: ______________ Date Tasted: ______

Region/Country: ______________

Grape: ______________

% Alcohol: ______________

Producer: __________ Vintage: __________

Importer/Distributor: __________

Price: __________

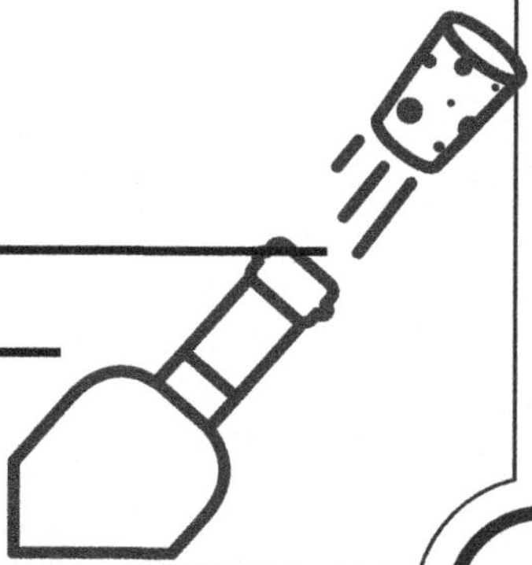

Color/Style: Red White Rose' Sparkling Effervescent Fortified

Appearance: Thin Thick

Dry/Sweet Spectrum: Dry 1 2 3 4 5 6 7 8 9 10 Sweet

Body: Light Light to Medium Medium Medium to Full Full Overall

Tasting Experience: Poor 1 2 3 4 5 6 7 8 9 10 Excellent

Comments:

____

____

____

____

Recommended Not Recommended

Circle One

Made in the USA
Monee, IL
04 November 2026

67379933R00056